Evidence-Based Palliative Care Across The Life Span

Huda Huijer Abu-Saad

Professor of Nursing Science
Director, Centre for Nursing Research
Faculty of Health Sciences, Maastricht University

With contributions from

Annemie Courtens

Centre for Development of Palliative Care
University Hospital Maastricht

Blackwell
Science

© 2001 by
Blackwell Science Ltd
Editorial Offices:
Osney Mead, Oxford OX2 0EL
25 John Street, London WC1N 2BS
23 Ainslie Place, Edinburgh EH3 6AJ
350 Main Street, Malden
  MA 02148 5018, USA
54 University Street, Carlton
  Victoria 3053, Australia
10, rue Casimir Delavigne
  75006 Paris, France

Other Editorial Offices:

Blackwell Wissenschafts-Verlag GmbH
Kurfürstendamm 57
10707 Berlin, Germany

Blackwell Science KK
MG Kodenmacho Building
7–10 Kodenmacho Nihombashi
Chuo-ku, Tokyo 104, Japan

Iowa State University Press
A Blackwell Science Company
2121 S. State Avenue
Ames, Iowa 50014-8300, USA

First published 2001

Set in 10/12.5 Sabon
by DP Photosetting, Aylesbury, Bucks

DISTRIBUTORS

Marston Book Services Ltd
PO Box 269
Abingdon
Oxon OX14 4YN
(*Orders:* Tel: 01235 465500
            Fax: 01235 465555)

USA
Blackwell Science, Inc.
Commerce Place
350 Main Street
Malden, MA 02148 5018
(*Orders:* Tel: 800 759 6102
            781 388 8250
            Fax: 781 388 8255)

Canada
Login Brothers Book Company
324 Saulteaux Crescent
Winnipeg, Manitoba R3J 3T2
(*Orders:* Tel: 204 837-2987
            Fax: 204 837-3116)

Australia
Blackwell Science Pty Ltd
54 University Street
Carlton, Victoria 3053
(*Orders:* Tel: 03 9347 0300
            Fax: 03 9347 5001)

A catalogue record for this title is available from
the British Library

ISBN 0-632-05818-8

Library of Congress
Cataloging-in-Publication Data
Abu-Saad, Huda, 1949
    Evidence-based palliative care across the life
span/Huda Huijer Abu-Saad; with
contributions from Annemie Courtens.
    p. cm.
Includes bibliographical references and index.
ISBN 0-632-05818-8
1. Palliative treatment.   2. Evidence-based
medicine.
I. Courtens, Annemie.   II. Title.
R726.8 .A28 2001
616'.029–dc21

                                    00-052913

For further information on
Blackwell Science, visit our website:
www.blackwell-science.com

Contents

Foreword

Palliative care is the technical term for comfort care at the end of life. It is appropriate when efforts to prevent death (and thereby prolong life) become increasingly futile. The focus moves from disease-control to patient-support and the quality of the person's remaining life. 'Palliative' is derived from *pallium*, the Latin word for cloak, and reflects the fact that, when the underlying disease cannot be cured, it is often possible to 'cloak' the symptoms – such as by 'cloaking' pain with analgesics and so on. A quotation from the Qu'ran, however, provides palliative care with a more poignant and profound meaning: 'May you be wrapped in tenderness, you my brother, as if in a cloak'.

There have always been people who have sensitively assisted those struggling to make sense of life in the midst of progressive and ultimately fatal disease. What is new, however, is the fact that many of us today have been enlightened and empowered through contact with modern palliative care teams, and further encouraged and supported by organisations such as the European Association for Palliative Care. A critical mass of enthusiasm and knowledge has been achieved and what, in past decades, was extraordinary and occasional is now received wisdom and clinical orthodoxy.

Although they are not the only way to deliver high quality care, palliative care units abound in the UK and are found increasingly elsewhere. The thought of a 'terminal care unit' elicits a mixture of responses. However, for most people, actually visiting one results in the strange discovery of life and joy in the midst of death and distress. It is in this paradox that the secret of palliative care resides, a paradox which is the end result of ordinary down-to-earth activities such as skilled nursing care, good symptom management and sensitive psychological support. In other words, human compassion in action. All are expressions of respect for the patient as a person and of corporate activity in which professional individualism is balanced by multiprofessional teamwork. The house of hospice model (Fig. F.1) is a good way of expressing this, with its foundation stones of acceptance ('Whatever happens, we will not abandon you') and affirmation ('You may be dying but you are important to us'). Hope, openness and honesty are the cement which holds the house together.

Indeed, globally, the biggest challenge facing doctors in relation to palliative care is the question of truthfulness with patients. It is still often said that telling patients that they are terminally ill destroys hope and leads to irreversible despair and depression. In reality the opposite is more often the case – lying and evasion isolate patients behind either a wall of words or a wall of silence which prevents

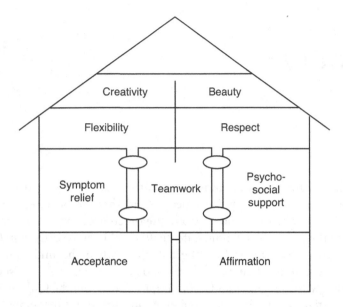

Fig. F.1   The house of hospice.

them from sharing their fears and anxieties. It is not possible to be hopeful in palliative care without a prior commitment to openness and honesty.

Palliative care acknowledges and responds to two levels of experience – the surface and the deep, the conscious and the unconscious, the tangible and the intangible (Kearney 1996). Activities which facilitate the crossing from the surface to the deep levels of experience are an important part of palliative care programmes – creative activity (poetry, art, crafts, etc.), music, massage, reminiscence and relaxation. The focus is on the search for meaning and making sense of the suffering.

This leads to difficulties in evaluation and the bureaucratically unsatisfactory conclusion that all that can be measured is not relevant and much that is relevant is not measurable. Whether this will always be so is debatable. Nonetheless, those working in specialist palliative care settings will be grateful to Professor Dr Abu-Saad and Dr Courtens for reviewing the different ways in which palliative care is presently delivered and examining the many questions surrounding its evaluation. This book will be an invaluable literary companion for policy makers, administrators, students, practitioners and researchers alike.

Palliative care is now accepted as important in an increasing number of countries by governmental health departments and by health professionals. Acceptance by the establishment leads to routinization and bureaucracy – which can stifle charisma and innovation. Palliative care needs to be both accepted and innovative. The final goal has not yet been reached. There is still a long way to go before all who need it receive high quality palliative care. Hence, the challenge for palliative care in the twenty-first century is to achieve a creative tension between stable bureaucracy and unstable charisma. Only by so doing will palliative care remain patient-focused whole-person care – adding life to people's days rather than days to people's lives.

Robert Twycross
Macmillan Clinical Reader in Palliative Medicine,
Oxford University;
Consultant Physician,
St Michael Sobel House, Oxford

Chapter 1

Introduction

Huda Huijer Abu-Saad

1.1 Introduction

In the last few decades of the twentieth century palliative care witnessed an explosion both in knowledge and in the provision of services in many countries worldwide. In many ways this process of expansion and proliferation is similar to the ongoing developments in clinical practice and health care policy. Many areas of clinical practice and in this case palliative care have seen an increased emphasis not only on patient-centred care, multidisciplinary collaboration, adequate co-ordination of care, and the provision of continuity of care, but also on expanding the boundaries of health care professionals involved in the care process. In addition, increased emphasis has been placed on the use of highly skilled nursing care as well as the appropriate psychosocial and complementary therapies in providing palliative care services. Similar developments have been witnessed at the social policy level. There is more emphasis placed on the quality of care provided and in particular on effectiveness and efficiency. Palliative care services face as a result the same demands as any other health care services for evidence of efficacy and cost-effectiveness.

The expansion in the type of health care services and the creation of expanded roles for health care professionals have persisted over the years without proper evaluation of their effectiveness. Many forms of quality assurance and audits have consequently become increasingly important and more emphasis has been placed recently on evaluation research to address questions of effectiveness and efficiency. The pressure from policy-makers is not limited to demonstrating the effectiveness of innovations in the health care services sector, but also extends to evaluating medical and health-related procedures. These pressures stem from a perceived need to use health care funds in the most efficient and effective way.

The extent to which palliative care has been evaluated is the focus of this book. The driving force behind undertaking such a task is the conviction of the authors that such a broad review of the developments in this area is worthwhile and much needed. The recognition that there is an established need for such a study in the field of palliative care provided enough incentive for the Pain Expertise Centre of the Academic Hospital in Maastricht to fund the preliminary part of this project, for which we are deeply grateful. The main purpose of this book is to provide an overview of the state of the art in palliative care across the life span. More specifically, the book addresses the following questions:

- Which types of palliative care models are currently in use for adults and children?
- What is the established evidence on effectiveness of palliative care models in use for adults and children?
- Which views do home carers and professional carers hold regarding palliative care?
- What is the extent of symptom prevalence and management in the palliative care of adults and children?
- Which instruments are currently developed and used in palliative care research?
- Which problems and pitfalls are encountered in palliative care research?
- How can the implementation of established evidence be facilitated in palliative care practices?

1.2   Methods

In conducting this state-of-the-art work, the intention was to identify all relevant literature in this area. To do so, an extensive search strategy was adopted. A Medline on-line literature search for the years 1980–2000 was carried out. The keywords used for this search were 'palliative care', 'care models', 'terminal illness', 'hospice care', 'pain and symptom management', 'quality of life', 'children', and 'evaluation of care'. Abstracts published in the abstract book of the congress of the European Association for Palliative Care were also used. Citations in identified articles were also screened and appropriate references accordingly used. The snowball method was also utilised to trace published articles. Articles in English, French, Dutch and German were included when possible.

Although there was a clear intention to include all possible scientific references published in this area, there is a possibility that a number of articles could not be traced, that the search was incomplete, and that the keywords used were not comprehensive enough to cover this vast and growing area. Taking these limitations into consideration, the authors believe that this review nevertheless provides the clinician and researcher in palliative care with a broad overview of the developments in this field up to the time of writing.

1.3   Chapter structure

The results of this state-of-the-art work are presented in 11 chapters. This first chapter provides a brief introduction, lists the research questions addressed, and describes the methods used in searching the literature. Chapter 2 gives an overview of the developments in palliative care. Chapter 3 reviews the models cited in the literature as used in palliative care in adults in different countries in the world.

Chapter 4 focuses on issues related to palliative care services in children. In Chapter 5 emphasis is placed on the effectiveness of palliative care models in use. Chapter 6 addresses views of home carers and health professionals with regard to palliative care services. Chapters 7 and 8 cover briefly the most prevalent symptoms in adults and children respectively. The effectiveness of specific management techniques for a number of symptoms is evaluated. This is not intended to be exhaustive in nature but rather exemplary. Symptom management constitutes by itself a topic for a special review and thus needs to be addressed more extensively elsewhere. Chapter 9 gives an overview of instruments used to assess the quality of palliative care. Emphasis is placed on quality of life, functional status and quality of care. Chapter 10 provides a critical analysis of the problems and pitfalls in palliative care research and makes recommendations for choice of designs and for future topics where research is still warranted. Finally, Chapter 11 ends the book by providing insight into the facilitating factors for implementing evidence in palliative care practices and reflects on the challenges facing palliative care in the future.

Chapter 2

Developments in Palliative Care

Huda Huijer Abu-Saad and Annemie Courtens

2.1 Introduction

This chapter gives, first, an overview of the history of palliative care. The most commonly used definitions are discussed next. The philosophy of palliative care and its distinguishing characteristics and objectives follow. Finally, attention is given to the founding of the European Association for Palliative Care and to its mission with regard to developments in this growing field of care.

2.2 The history of palliative care

The practice of palliative care resulted from the modern hospice movement about 30 years ago. Palliative care was, however, already provided in the ancient hospices, which originally arose in the fourth century. In the Eastern Mediterranean areas, prior to Christianity, sick people did not have places of extended care such as hospitals. Most of the care took place within the family. Phipps (1988) writes that the beginnings of hospitals relate to the Christian remembrance of the life and teachings of Jesus. According to Cohen (1979), the first hospitals (*hospitia*) were an offshoot of religion rather than of medicine. The first Christian emperor Constantine, for example, decreed in AD 335 the founding of *nosocomeia* (infirmaries) throughout the Roman empire (Canones Arabici Nicaeni 75, cited in Phipps, 1988). Centuries later, *nosocomeia* later called *hospitia* (Latin) could be found in many cities in the Mediterranean area.

Etymologically, the Latin word *hospitium* signifies 'the warm feeling between host and guest' or 'the place where the warm feeling between host and guest is experienced'. The French translation of *hospitium* is hospice, a term still used. The Benedictines in the sixth century were noted for their hospices. In them monks cared for pilgrims, often fatigued and exhausted. Gradually, though, the hospices gave refuge to the sick as well (Goldin, 1981). The terminally ill too found a resting place in the hospices. Before the Reformation many hospices were in existence throughout Europe, but during the Reformation many of them were closed. In monastic hospitals/hospices, the practice of medicine was elementary and the patient was cared for palliatively, providing food, warmth and kindness, and religious services which soothed when cure was not possible (Leff, 1956).

During the Protestant Reformation, the support of monasteries weakened. Secular rulers and physician groups gradually took over some of the services that hospices/hospitals provided.

In later centuries hospitals developed rapidly, becoming centres of cure. Care in an era of growing medical technology did not receive much attention, which led to a decrease in the holistic care given by the earlier hospitals/hospices (Phipps, 1987 cited in Phipps, 1988). Recognising the need for more patient-centred care attending to spiritual as well as physical needs of patients, more Christian-sponsored medical centres were erected in the twentieth century (Barret, 1982). Simultaneously, medical technology advanced rapidly which resulted in the generally accepted conception that patients had to be cured if possible. This conception strongly influenced the care of terminally ill patients. With the emphasis placed on cure, there was no room to discuss fears and concerns. Communication between patient, staff and family often ceased abruptly (Schneider *et al.*, 1996). Furthermore no priority was given to pain and symptom control, which was also the case for spiritual matters and anticipatory grieving. An integrated, more patient-centred approach was needed. The lack of adequate assessment and treatment of the physical and psychosocial problems of the terminally ill and their families led to new ideas concerning the balance between cure and care (Bruera, 1996).

During the 1960s the first steps were taken in the UK towards the development of modern palliative care (Bruera *et al.*, 1994a). The advocates of a holistic and more patient-centred approach were Dr. Cicely Saunders and Elisabeth Kübler Ross (Schneider *et al.*, 1996). Dr. Saunders emphasised the following objectives of care: care of the patient and family as a unit, an interdisciplinary team approach, the use of volunteers, a continuum of care that included the home setting, and follow-up of family members after the patient's death. This led to the opening of St Christopher's Hospice in London in 1967 by Dr Saunders. The first steps in the modern hospice movement were taken, giving the philosophy of hospice/palliative care a chance to develop further in, for example, Great Britain and the USA. Elisabeth Kübler Ross' book *On Death and Dying*, published in 1969, brought about a new discussion of death and dying, topics that had been avoided for an era, and prepared the ground for the growth of hospice home-care teams in the United States (Schonwetter, 1996; Doyle *et al.*, 1998). Hospice in the USA became a concept of care rather than a place of care. During the 1970s the United States, in contrast with Great Britain, delivered hospice care in the patient's own home, if at all possible, thus responding to the patient's wish to die at home (Schonwetter, 1996; Von Gunten *et al.*, 1996). The term palliative care was gradually brought into the lexicon as a synonym of hospice care. In Canada a Palliative Care Service was opened in the Royal Victoria Hospital in 1975 in Montreal (Waller, 1996).

The period from the 1970s to the 1990s brought about an expansion of palliative care programmes in the UK, in Europe and in North America. The number of hospices increased to about 700 in the UK and 1500 in the USA (Waller, 1996). Palliative care programmes also developed in the 1990s in Australia, Asia (mainly in Japan, South Korea, Taiwan and China) and in African countries like Zimbabwe and South Africa (Martinson, 1996). International congresses are held on palliative care to share experiences and research findings in the developing field of palliative care. National and international organisations such as the European Association for Palliative Care or the National Hospice Organisation in the USA are established to exchange knowledge and experiences among the disciplines involved in palliative care. Moreover, several journals on palliative care are currently published, a number of textbooks in palliative medicine and palliative care have been written, and chairs in palliative medicine have been established at universities in the UK, Canada and Australia (Waller, 1996).

2.3 Definition

The term 'palliative' comes from the Latin word *pallium*, which means 'cloak' or 'cover'. Symbolically, palliative care can be a cloak of warmth and protection given to the terminally ill patients by their caregivers (Francke *et al.*, 1997). Twycross (1997) states: 'In palliative care the symptoms are "cloaked" with treatments whose primary and sole aim is to promote patient comfort.' In the 16th century the term 'palliative' was first used in medicine to describe alleviation or mitigation of suffering (George & Jennings, 1993). This definition has survived the centuries and is still being used. In the modern hospice movement, palliation was defined originally as: 'The management of patients in whom death is almost certain and not too far off, where the control of symptoms is the prime clinical objective and the emotional and spiritual preparation of both patients and "family" is given high priority' (Holford, 1973 cited in George & Jennings, 1993).

The first definition of 'palliative medicine' was in 1987, coinciding with the acceptance of palliative medicine in the UK as a formal medical speciality (Doyle *et al.*, 1998). The definition states that: 'Palliative medicine is the study and management of patients with active, progressive, and far-advanced disease for whom the prognosis is limited and the focus of care is quality of life.' This definition places emphasis on the terminal character of the disease. In later definitions the concept of palliative care was broadened to include the area of life-threatening disease too (Higginson, 1993).

In a palliative care team in which doctors, nurses, therapists, social workers, clergy and volunteers are involved, palliative care as defined by the European Association of Palliative Care (George & Jennings, 1993) or the World Health Organisation (WHO, 1990) seems more appropriate. The definition stated by the European Association of Palliative Care involves:

> 'The provision of active total care when disease is not responsive to curative treatment. Palliative care neither hastens nor postpones death; provides relief from pain and other distressing symptoms; integrates the psychological and spiritual aspects of care and offers a support system to help the family cope during the patients' illness and in bereavement.'

The WHO (1990) defines palliative care as:

'the active total care of patients whose disease is not responsive to curative treatment. Control of pain, of other symptoms, and of psychological, social and spiritual problems is paramount. The goal of palliative care is achievement of the best possible quality of life for patients and their families. Many aspects of palliative care are applicable earlier in the course of the illness, in conjunction with anticancer treatment'.
(In this report, 'family' refers to either actual relatives or other key people.)

By way of further explaining the definition, WHO (1990) provides guiding principles that indicate that:

'palliative care:

(1) Affirms life and regards dying as a normal process;
(2) Neither hastens nor postpones death;
(3) Provides relief from pain and other distressing symptoms;
(4) Integrates the psychological and spiritual aspects of patient care;
(5) Offers a support system to help patients live as actively as possible until death;
(6) Offers a support system to help the family cope during the patient's illness and in their own bereavement.'

Twycross (1997) defines palliative care as follows:

'Palliative care is the active total care of patients and their families by a multiprofessional team at a time when the patient's disease is no longer responsive to curative treatment and life expectancy is relatively short. It responds to physical, psychological, social and spiritual needs, and extends if necessary to support in bereavement.'

Considering the above-mentioned definitions of palliative care of the 1990s, it seems that the definition of the European Association of Palliative Care (George & Jennings, 1993) and the WHO (1990) definition formed the basis for the definitions which originated later (Burucoa, 1991; Francke *et al.*, 1997; Steiner, 1997; Twycross, 1997). The WHO definition differs in some aspects from the definition of the European Association of Palliative Care, by including the aspects 'palliative care affirms life and regards dying as a normal process' and correspondingly 'palliative care offers a support system to help patients live as actively as possible until death'. These aspects accentuate the quality of life remaining for the dying persons and emphasise their well being. Twycross broadens the definition of palliative care by integrating the concepts of a 'multiprofessional team', 'life expectancy' and 'bereavement support'. The 'patient's family' is accentuated and gets special attention with regard to the active total care needed. Twycross (1997) extends further the fourth and fifth WHO guiding principles to include:

- 'Integrating psychological, social and spiritual aspects of care so that patients may come to terms with their own death as fully and constructively as they can.'
- 'Offering a support system to help patients live as actively and creatively as possible until death.'

In conclusion, the practice of palliative care is considered in most definitions to integrate the psycho (emotional), social, physical (biological) and spiritual aspects of care. In all definitions of palliative care emphasis is placed more on relieving suffering and providing comfort and less on curing the disease.

2.4   Philosophy of palliative care

Palliative care may be regarded to have evolved from the hospice objectives, being founded on the same philosophical thoughts (Rousseau, 1995). The philosophy of palliative care is expressed briefly in the definitions of palliative care stated earlier (NHO, 1993; Johnston & Abraham, 1995; Leland & Schonwetter, 1997). Leland & Schonwetter (1997) add three new philosophical ideas with specific relevance to hospice care: 'bereavement care to friends', 'care provision regardless of ability to pay', as well as the use of an 'interdisciplinary team'. In general, however, the philosophy of palliative care encompasses two major goals: effective symptom control and maintenance of quality of life. With the purpose of achieving those philosophical goals, a multi- or interdisciplinary team (Ajemian, 1993; Leland & Schonwetter, 1997) is needed with the unit of care being the patient and his family.

Interdisciplinary team

Prior to discussing the use of an interdisciplinary team within the philosophy of palliative care, the differences between multi- and interdisciplinary palliative care need to be clarified. In a multidisciplinary team, the professional identity of the team members is usually subordinate to the team affiliation. The multi-disciplinary team knows one professional who is highest in rank, and care is evaluated on the basis of the patient's medical record. Thus interaction between the team members can be regarded as of secondary importance. In the inter-disciplinary team, the identity of the professionals is superseded by the identity of the team. The different team members, depending on the task at hand, assume leadership in the team. In order to develop goals, information is shared among team members and the work is done interdependently.

The interdisciplinary team can be considered as a vehicle of action in which the interaction process is vital to success. Negotiation and discussion form the basic elements of an interdisciplinary team, each team member willing to consider the viewpoint of the others (Lowe, 1981; Ajemian, 1993; Doyle *et al.*, 1998). In spite of these theoretical distinctions between a multidisciplinary and an inter-disciplinary team, in practice both types of team display overlapping functions.

Negotiations and discussions about the needs of the patient and with regard to providing quality palliative care become of primary importance. Only in sharing information regarding the patient's constitution and relevant to the care needed, can an interdisciplinary team provide holistic palliative care to the terminally ill patient (Cassel, 1991).

Patient and family – a unit of care

In palliative care the patient is considered in a wider context and the provision of care is centred on the patient and his family who are considered to be the unit of care. Investigations, procedures and treatments on behalf of the patient have to be carried out at a cost/benefit ratio in favour of the patient. Furthermore, the individuality of the patient must be taken into account, which can be achieved by involving the patient in decisions concerning the provision of care. In these decisions it is also important to involve the patient's family as the patient and family are regarded to be the unit of care (Twycross, 1991; Connolly, 1994). Active involvement of the patient in the decision-making process provides a mechanism in which the patient's rights for a good, dignified and graceful death are respected (George, 1991).

Viewing the patient and his family as the unit of care requires a holistic approach in palliative care. Holism according to Dicks (1989) is 'seeing people as a whole; the person, not the disease or the symptoms being the focus of treatment'. Dicks (1989) states further that from a holistic point of view the individual is allowed to take as much responsibility for himself and his health as he wants to. In palliative care where the emphasis is on the short term, this is of particular importance.

Difference between palliative and hospice care

Hospice care and palliative care share the same philosophy mentioned earlier. Hospice care, however, cannot be considered similar to palliative care. Portenoy (1996) states that palliative care may differ from hospice care on the following grounds:

- 'Care provision concerning the comfort and functioning of patients and their families at all stages of disease,
- Strong physician input on an ongoing basis,
- Willingness to use aggressive "tertiary" interventions such as primary anticancer therapies and invasive treatments of symptom control for appropriate patients,
- Acceptance of research for quality improvement and scientific advancement.'

Furthermore, Portenoy (1996) writes, 'the palliative care model is appropriate for patients with any life-threatening disease during and after the period of aggressive primary therapy'.

Palliative care when not provided at the end-stage of the life-threatening disease can be a mixture of symptom management, function-oriented therapies, and psychosocial support and interventions. In the terminal stage of the disease, palliative care is usually delivered following the hospice principles.

Care or cure in palliative care

Palliative care is oriented to patients who are incurable. This is often about people who are going to die soon, although this will not always be the case. Often patients are confronted with a phase in which they know that cure is not possible, but death is not yet approaching them (Spreeuwenberg, 1997). The phase in which there are no possibilities left for cure could last for weeks, months and sometimes several years (COPZ, 1998). The illness being either incurable or not treatable due to a pre-existing iatrogenic morbidity, can shift the patient's orientation from quantity of life to quality of life (George & Jennings, 1993).

In palliative care the balance between caring and curing is sometimes difficult to find. According to the palliative care ideology, there is an appropriate moment in the course of the illness when the goal must change from curing to caring. With quality of life becoming paramount, the accent shifts from the disease to the patient and family (Friel, 1982; WHO, 1990; Rousseau, 1995).

In the conventional model of treating patients with life-threatening disease, care can be divided into three phases: curative, palliative and terminal.

The curative phase is the phase where cure or complete remission of the disease is still a possible expectation. The aim of care is survival of the patient. In this phase the management of the disease process is dominant; treatment-related toxicity and morbidity are accepted (Ashby & Stofell, 1991)

The second phase is the phase where curative treatment is no longer expected to prolong life. The aim of treatment in this phase is to maximise the quality of life of the patient by promoting his capacities to make and take responsibility for his own choices. Treatment side effects should be less harmful than the effects of cancer itself (Ashby & Stofell, 1991). The balance of curative treatment to prolong life versus palliative treatment is directed to comfort measures, symptom relief and common well being.

The third phase, in which there is clinical evidence of a dying process and bereavement, can be called the terminal phase. At this time all measures which are not required for comfort are withdrawn and treatment toxicity is no longer accepted. Harmful or distressing side effects are not acceptable. The aim of care is to die with dignity.

At first glance, it seems that this conventional model of care of patients with life-threatening disease may be divided into different phases, each determined by the primary goal of treatment: curative, palliative and terminal. This model suggests that the boundaries between these phases are clear and the focus of change is the progression of disease pathology.

Jeffrey (1995) examined this model and concluded that the boundaries between these phases of care are blurred and that the divisions between the phases are artificial. The timing of the change from a curative to palliative approach to caring is a complex clinical and moral dilemma, which is fundamental to the care of patients (Jeffrey, 1995). Delay in making the decision to change may result in a patient receiving inappropriate therapy designed to maintain hope rather than offer a chance of prolonged remission or cure. On the other hand physicians do not want to stand accused of neglecting patients when further curative treatments might be possible (Jeffrey, 1995). These dilemmas will lead to uncertainties among physicians, nurses, patients and their relatives.

According to Jeffrey (1995) the key to coping with these uncertainties which arise in beginning and ending palliative care lies in the process of sharing information and respecting patient autonomy. Doctors need to share their uncertainty with patients and families and with their nursing colleagues. Only by sharing information can they determine what choice to make.

Currently, palliative care is more and more seen as a continuum (see Fig. 2.1). The curative, palliative and terminal phases are not distinguished in a strict way. Comfort and supportive treatment are initiated when symptoms present themselves and continue with greater or lesser intensity until the final phase of life, at which time the intensity increases. Early interventions aimed at managing prevalent problems during the early stages of the disease may prevent symptom exacerbation, thus leading to decreased levels of distress and discomfort. Specialist palliative care units emphasise the importance of early referral of patients if the highest standards of care are to be achieved. This model also implicates that there is a role for disease specific therapy in palliative care. For example, radiotherapy may be advocated for use in the last phase of life if the purpose of the therapy is to provide symptom control. In this model bereavement support is seen as an integral part of palliative care.

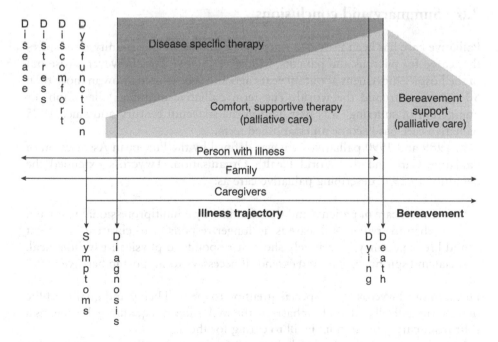

Fig. 2.1 The continuum of palliative care (Doyle *et al.*, 1998).

2.5   European Association for Palliative Care

The European Association for Palliative Care (EAPC) was created in 1991 by 42 founding members from nine European countries. EAPC development reflects the rapid growth of palliative care in Europe. The association is actually a federation of organisations and an association with individual members. By the end of 1995, the association had, in addition to individual membership, ten collective national associations as members, which together add up to around 8000 members from 28 European countries and 24 non-European countries. An increment of 4000 members is also foreseen in the near future. In addition to formal connections with national associations, the EAPC has established liaisons with the International Association for the Study of Pain (IASP), the World Health Organisation (WHO), and the European School of Oncology.

EAPC maintains updated directories of persons involved and interested in palliative care, of organisations and associations in palliative care, and of official documents on subjects regarding palliative care. In addition, the EAPC organises biennial congresses as well as expert meetings on controversial aspects of palliative care. The EAPC has in addition a review journal, the *European Journal of Palliative Care* (EJPC), and a newsletter that is circulated to caregivers interested in palliative care. The association has furthermore developed networks in the areas of education, ethics and research in palliative care which are aimed to facilitate further developments in these areas through collaborative efforts at the European and international levels.

2.6   Summary and conclusions

Palliative care has been provided since the beginning of Christianity in hospices that cared for pilgrims and patients. Modern palliative care, however, arose out of the hospice movement about 30 years ago and is developing now in more than 50 countries around the world. The term palliative meaning 'alleviation' or 'mitigation of suffering' was first used in the sixteenth century and since 1975 palliative care has become an established term.

In 1989 and 1990 palliative care was defined by the European Association of Palliative Care and the World Health Organisation. Twycross extended the definition in 1997 describing palliative care as:

> 'active total care of patients and their families by a multiprofessional team at a time when the patient's disease is no longer responsive to curative treatment and life expectancy is relatively short. It responds to physical, psychological, social and spiritual needs, and extends if necessary to support in bereavement.'

Furthermore Twycross gave special attention to the well being and quality of life of the terminally ill patient. Emphasising the well being and quality of life means a shift from curing the terminally ill to caring for them.

In the course of the terminal disease curative and palliative care are not mutually exclusive. The philosophical ideologies in palliative care emphasise the importance of maintaining a balance between care and cure. Other relevant aspects of palliative care within the same philosophy include giving attention to 'multi- or interdisciplinary team work' and to considering 'patient and family as the unit of care'. Finally, the provision of high quality care, within a holistic framework, necessitates the involvement of the patient and family in decisions concerning diagnostic work and treatments. This is the only way that the patient can be assured of a good death with dignity and respect.

Chapter 3

Models of Palliative Care

Huda Huijer Abu-Saad and Annemie Courtens

3.1 Introduction

Palliative care can be provided intramurally and extramurally to patients with terminal illnesses. Several models of care in domiciliary, inpatient and outpatient/consultative settings have been developed over the last 30 years to provide palliative care in about 50 countries in the world. In the UK, the USA and the Netherlands most of these models have been put into practice (Francke *et al.*, 1997; Twycross, 1997; Doyle *et al.*, 1998). Several European countries such as Scandinavia, Ireland, France, Germany, Italy, Spain, Switzerland, Austria, Poland, Slovakia and Greece are developing palliative care programmes too (Luczak, 1993; Maddocks, 1993; Ventafridda *et al.*, 1993; Blumhuber *et al.* 1996; Klaschik & Husebo, 1997; Mercadante *et al.*, 1997; Sadovska, 1997; Steiner, 1997). Furthermore, other parts of the world like Australia, New Zealand and some Asian, African and South American countries recognise the importance of palliative care and are already providing palliative care services to some extent (Wenk, 1993; Martinson, 1996; Dwyer, 1997). In this chapter, special emphasis is given to palliative care models in the UK, the USA and the Netherlands.

3.2 Palliative care models

Palliative care can be provided in domiciliary, inpatient and outpatient settings, as well as through day care and consultation services. In domiciliary settings, palliative home care is delivered in most countries by well-established primary health care facilities. The care is mostly provided by a general practitioner with or without community nurses (Doyle *et al.*, 1998). Inpatient settings include hospices or homes for the terminally ill, general or specialised units in (specialised) hospitals or nursing homes, (specialised) homes for the elderly and homes for terminally ill children. Patients who are able to visit the hospital can receive care from a specialist palliative care outpatient unit or from a consultation service (Keating, 1996; Schonwetter, 1996; Doyle *et al.*, 1998). Furthermore, hospices or specialised units in hospitals provide day care for terminally ill patients. Most of these services operate on weekdays from 10 AM. to 4 PM. One of the most inter-

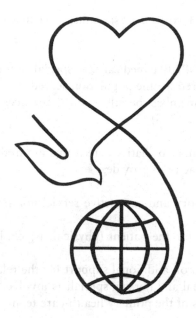

Fig. 3.1 Globe of care. (Courtesy of Simon Andras, Budapest)

esting and important developments in the provision of specialist palliative care is the emergence of hospital-based palliative care teams or symptom relief teams. Despite being an advisory service to other caregivers, these teams are able to provide facilities for effective symptom control, which enables patients to spend more time at home.

Domiciliary services

In the UK, the USA and the Netherlands, the primary health care team is of major importance in the care of the terminally ill. The general practitioner has overall responsibility for the medical care of patients and the district nurses play a key role in nursing care. The general practitioner or nurse co-ordinates the care provided to terminally ill patients. Other disciplines involved in the care of patient and family are social workers, physiotherapists, chaplains, psychologists and volunteers. Nursing care in the UK is also provided by Marie Curie Cancer Nurses and Macmillan nurses. These nurses are specialists in cancer care and are responsible for providing symptom relief, psychosocial support, information and support in bereavement (Saunders, 1983; Kindlen, 1988; Garland, 1994; Webber, 1994).

When the patient needs specialist medical treatment or if more complex psychological problems develop, a referral by the general practitioner to hospital-based specialists or a clinical psychologist may be necessary.

In Great Britain the primary care teams are often supported by palliative care/ home care teams, which exist in most districts (Kindlen, 1988; Boyd, 1994;

O'Neill & Rodway, 1998). Two types of specialist domiciliary palliative services have been developed:

- A team consisting of a palliative medical care specialist and as many clinical nurse specialists as required for the population served
- An all-nurse team, each member specially trained and accredited in palliative nursing care (Doyle *et al.*, 1998).

The majority of the domiciliary palliative care teams are multiprofessional and function in an advisory capacity to provide:

- A complementary, advisory and supportive service for primary health-care teams
- Advice on all palliation for the patient (physical, psychological, social and spiritual)
- Advice on, and provision of, additional support for the relatives
- Liaison with other medical and nursing specialists involved in palliative care
- Support for the members of the primary health-care team.

Some of these teams operate 24 hours around the clock, others from 9 AM to 5 PM.

New types of domiciliary care have developed in the UK: rapid response teams and respite care teams. The rapid response team can be considered as an emergency 'crisis intervention' service which is called by a general practitioner/family doctor when the terminally ill patient at home is in a crisis. Rapid response teams include a medical palliative care specialist and nursing palliative care specialists, responding directly in a crisis situation. The team is expected to intervene and stay with the family until the situation has settled. Acute states of confusion, inexplicable pain or urgent suprapubic catheterisation are examples of crises necessitating rapid response team intervention. The respite care teams are called upon to relieve the family of the terminally ill patient for a few hours each day. This respite time can be used by the family to take care of chores left undone or as time off from their daily patient care routines (Doyle *et al.*, 1998).

In the USA palliative care at the patient's home is referred to as hospice home care. The growth of the hospice movement in the USA has been slower than in the UK for numerous reasons, like the differences between medical practice, education and patient expectations. However, over the last quarter of the twentieth century the hospice movement grew to a regulated approach reimbursed by Medicare and other insurance programmes. There are nearly 1900 hospice programmes in the USA (Plumb & Ogle, 1992). Most of these programmes place emphasis on home care. Community-based models are either freestanding units or offices that serve as co-ordinating points. These models arose from existing home care agencies or volunteer hospices. So-called 'back-up beds' are contracted through local hospitals or nursing homes (Plumb & Ogle, 1992).

The goals of home hospice care are to have the patient comfortable and able to deal with approaching death. Not only physical needs but emotional, spiritual, psychological and even financial and legal concerns are important (Rhymes,

1991).The patient's own general practitioner and the community nurses are the core team in providing palliative care to the patient and family, but other disciplines like the chaplain, therapists or social worker might be involved. The palliative care services are nurse co-ordinated (McNally *et al.*, 1996). A hospice medical director can provide consultation on pain and symptom control (Rhymes, 1991).

A core team consisting of the general practitioner and community nurses mostly provides palliative home care in the Netherlands. Sometimes specialised district nurses play an advisory role. The co-ordination of care is carried out either by the general practitioner or by a nurse. It is possible to receive care at night (night-sitting services) from nurses from what is called 'intensive home care'. Other disciplines that might be involved are physiotherapists, pastoral workers and volunteers. There are more than 140 locations where help from volunteers for terminal patients is organised (Francke *et al.*, 1997). Volunteers support the family with caring and household activities, give emotional support and sometimes stay with the family and patient at night. The tasks of the volunteers are complementary to the professional help from GPs and nurses. Many initiatives have been developed in order to enhance continuity of care for terminal patients (Francke *et al.*, 1997). So-called 'shared care' has been developed in 46 locations (Francke *et al.*, 1997), covering integrated or transmural care projects which include for example technological care (like pain treatment or infusion) at home, consultations at home by specialised nurses, or 24-hour services. Recently in some places multidisciplinary palliative care teams have been started in order to support the primary health care professionals at home (Centres for the Development of Palliative Care in the Terminal Phase (Francke *et al.*, 1997)).

Inpatient services

There are several different organisational models for inpatient services for palliative care. Palliative care is provided in hospices or homes for the terminally ill, in palliative care units in general or specialised hospitals, in nursing homes, and in homes for the elderly.

Hospices

The first modern hospices began to appear in the late 1960s and 1970s inspired by the pioneering work of St Christopher's in London. A hospice provides multidisciplinary team care that aims to meet the complex and changing needs of people with a life-threatening disease, and their family. Hospices might be separate, freestanding units within a hospital/nursing home complex or geographically independent. Hospices offer a wide range of care: symptom control, rehabilitation, terminal care, outpatient support, family counselling, day care and bereavement follow-up. A hospice team usually consists of nurses, doctors, therapists, social workers, a chaplain, volunteers and sometimes a psychologist or counsellor and various complementary therapists.

Hospices are to be found in almost every country of the Western World. In the UK one fifth of the hospices are run by National Health Trusts; others are wholly or partly funded by charity. In the USA the emphasis remains on home care but notable initiatives for hospices have been taken by major teaching hospitals (Doyle *et al.*, 1998). In the Netherlands 10 hospices exist, three of which are integrated in nursing homes, while the others are not integrated in regular care. The hospices have mostly a homely atmosphere; patients have a lot of privacy; there are also opportunities for relatives and friends to stay at night; and people can bring some of their own belongings. Plans and initiatives are underway to build four new hospices. The Dutch government is pushing, however, for the integration of hospices in regular care facilities such as nursing homes, homes for the elderly and hospitals.

Day care or day hospices

The broad aims of hospice day care include:

(1)   Maintaining or improving the client's quality of life
(2)   The provision of holistic care by a multiprofessional team
(3)   The opportunity for rehabilitation within disease constraints
(4)   The continuity of care through interdisciplinary and interinstitution collaboration
(5)   Helping patients to continue living at home for as long as they think it is possible.

(Spencer & Daniels 1998)

In several countries there are growing numbers of day care facilities for patients under domiciliary care. These units operate on weekdays for about six hours a day. People attending from home are brought and taken home by car. Most of these units are staffed by nurses, physiotherapists, occupational therapists and volunteers. Day care might be very supportive for patients in a certain stage of their illness, especially if they want to remain as independent as possible but need some help such as having a weekly bath. Day care is also a way of supporting carers or introducing a patient who lives alone to a hospice team before the time they may need terminal care. Many day units also provide the opportunities for patients to be creative, join in with group activities and remain as active as possible.

Palliative care units in hospitals

There are only a limited number of palliative care units in hospitals in the UK, which may be a result of the large number of hospices that were built as a result of the hospice movement. However, palliative units in hospitals are more popular in other countries like the USA and Canada, where the charitable sector has been less involved in setting up hospices (Dunlop & Hockley, 1998). In the Netherlands, one palliative unit exists in a specialist cancer centre and one in a general hospital. Palliative care provision in hospital units is advantaged compared to other inpatient services by having diagnostic and specialist consultation services at hand, such as oncologists or internists. All senior medical and nursing staff are appropriately qualified in palliative care. Besides medical and nursing staff, there might be physiotherapists, chaplains, social workers and occupational therapists involved in the care of terminally ill patients. Most units provide a homely atmosphere and background technology is kept to a minimum (Francke *et al.*, 1997; Teunissen & van den Blink, 1997; Dunlop & Hockley, 1998). Facilities are often available to allow relatives to stay overnight.

Nursing homes

Nursing homes are traditionally involved with the care of chronically ill or terminally ill patients. In the USA some nursing homes have a contract with a hospice programme. Medicare Hospice Benefit helps with many tasks involved with palliative management of nursing home residents who are identified as having a limited life expectancy, including hospice nursing care, social services, consultation by a hospice medical director, counselling services or pastoral care. Some nursing homes have special units that handle the care of the dying residents, but most facilities allow these residents to stay in their usual room (Keay & Schonwetter, 1998).

Castle *et al.* (1997) provide a comprehensive examination of this phenomenon in their study conducted in the USA. They show that being small, being a proprietary facility, being part of a chain, having high tech capacity and a high skill level of staffing mix, and being located in a competitive environment are significantly related to having a hospice special care unit. Research on nursing home hospice facilities will have important implications for future government funding in this area.

In the Netherlands there are 326 nursing homes. Looking at the place of death in 1996, 36% of the total number of 135 000 dying people in the Netherlands died in a hospital, 17% died in a nursing home, 16% in a home for the elderly and 30% at home. Nursing homes have a lot of experience in the provision of palliative care to patients who have non-malignant diseases, but are also very willing to develop short-term terminal care for cancer patients. Nine nursing homes with specialised palliative units were identified, but there are many initiatives to integrate hospice care in many other nursing homes (Francke *et al.*, 1997; Baar, 1999). In the specialised units patients who could not stay at home or in hospital are admitted. Almost all patients had advanced cancer and died within ten days (Bruntink, 1998). Twenty nursing homes are members of Platform Palliative Terminal Care. This platform has several objectives: sharing experiences, developing expertise and co-ordinating care in order to improve the quality of palliative care in nursing homes.

Palliative care teams

The hospital-based palliative care team is the most recent evolution of the hospice movement. The first hospital-based palliative team was established in St Luke's

Hospital in New York in 1975 (Dunlop & Hockley, 1998). In the UK St Thomas' Hospital in London started a team in 1976. There are now more than 240 palliative care teams in the various university and district general hospitals in the UK (Doyle *et al.*, 1998). All these teams use a multidisciplinary approach including several disciplines. In almost all palliative care teams clinical nurse specialists form the backbone of the service. One or more doctors, a social worker, a psychologist, a secretary and a member of the clergy may also be represented in many different combinations, as well as volunteers, bereavement counsellors and health visitors.

The teams have no dedicated beds of their own but respond to invitations from departments (doctors/nurses) in the hospitals. The team has mostly an advisory role and is able to facilitate a level of symptom control, which enables patients to be discharged to home earlier. Most of the teams also have a teaching role, with team members teaching in medical and nursing schools. The palliative care team within the acute setting can also be a bridge to hospice home care services or hospice service.

In the Netherlands six palliative care teams started in 1999 with a project grant from the Dutch government. Some of the teams initiated in these projects are hospital-based; others work in the community while some work in both settings (Centres of Development of Palliative Care (Francke *et al.*, 1997)). All these multidisciplinary teams have an advisory and teaching role towards professional caregivers and/or patients. Some of the teams only do consultations by telephone while others also perform bedside consultations. The palliative care teams will be evaluated within two years in order to choose the best team model. The six centres for development of palliative care together developed a registration form, which constitutes the basis for this evaluation.

These projects fit into the stimulation programme of the Dutch Ministry of Health, which funded six centres for the development of palliative care in Amsterdam, Rotterdam, Utrecht, Groningen, Nijmegen and Maastricht. The centres are collaborations of universities, academic hospitals, comprehensive cancer centres and other institutions. All these centres are encouraged to improve palliative care by means of research, education of professionals, introduction of new care models and networking. The Dutch government is trying to base its policy of palliative care on research into needs of patients and families, epidemiological data and the evaluation of care models.

3.3   Members of an interdisciplinary palliative care team

Chronic life-limiting illness is characterised by complex and multidimensional suffering. Multidimensional suffering is best addressed through the investment of an interdisciplinary team that includes medical and non-medical health care disciplines.

Interdisciplinary collaboration in palliative care serves to realise the values expressed by the patient and the family and at the same time emphasises the values of the team involved in palliative care and their emphasis on excellence and effectiveness (Coyle, 1997). The goal of interdisciplinary palliative care is the provision of excellent care taking into consideration the complexity of care provided, the utilisation of the appropriate skills provided by the interprofessional team members, and the minimisation of fragmentation of care. Some of the requirements for collaborative practice include a clear definition of the skills, roles and education of each team member, defining the attributes of team members, commitment to a set of goals, defining the channels of communication within and outside the team, and defining the methods to enhance team cohesion and support.

It has been suggested that the dynamic of an interdisciplinary team is one of mutuality (we are all in this together), respect (what you bring to the healing dynamic is just as important as what I bring), and interdependence (if participation by any of us is hindered, healing will be hindered). Coyle (1997) lists a number of barriers in implementing collaborative palliative care services: the culture of the institution such as the hierarchical authority of the physician in relation to nurse, the issues regarding 'ownership of the patient', and the question of expertise with regard to profession, service and team. Another study described the factors which can weaken the vision to establish a team and threaten its survival; lack of funding or commitment at executive board level, failure in communication, and confusion about the different roles and skills of team members were mentioned. Sometimes the boundaries between roles of team members are less defined.

In the majority of palliative care teams, clinical nurse specialists form the backbone of the service. One or more physicians, a social worker, a psychologist, the clergy or volunteers may work as an integral part of some teams. Below, the roles of the nurse, the physician, the social worker and clergy are described.

The role of the nurse

In many ways the role of the nurse in the interdisciplinary palliative care team is more blurred than for other team members. This is partly because of the skills nurses should have in symptom control and psychosocial care but also because of the intuitive learned experience of nursing dying patients and their families in general (Dunlop & Hockley, 1998)

Dunlop and Hockley stated that one of the nurses in a palliative care team must be confident and skilled in the area of difficult symptom control in order to enable nurses on the team to undertake advisory and teaching roles. Both informal and formal teaching should represent a significant proportion of the role. In a study conducted by Davies and Oberle (1990), the role of the nurse in palliative care was investigated. Data were derived based on in-depth interviews with nurses working in an interdisciplinary team. The results showed that the role of the nurse can be defined as a supportive one with multiple dimensions: valuing, connecting, empowering, doing for, finding meaning and preserving own integrity. Valuing emphasises having respect for the inherent worth. Connecting denotes getting in touch with patient and family and entering their experience. Empowering refers to enabling the patient and family to do things for themselves and to do whatever they can to meet their own needs. Doing for focuses on the other hand on the physical care of the patient; it focuses on enabling the patient to use his or her own resources in controlling pain and other symptoms. In palliative care the nurse helps the patient in finding meaning to the present situation which is also strength giving and empowering. Finally, the nurse needs to preserve her own integrity by maintaining her self-esteem, self-worth and energy levels in order to function effectively. Clearly the concept of support forms the basis for understanding the knowledge and skills required of the nurse to function in such a setting and to be able to fulfil such a demanding role.

Dobratz (1990) defines the role of the palliative care nurse to include intensive caring, collaborative sharing, continuous knowing and continuous giving. Intensive caring involves the effective management of the physical, psychological, social and spiritual problems of patients and their families. Collaborative sharing incorporates the co-ordination of the care in a collaborative and interdisciplinary manner. Continuous knowing emphasises the continuous acquisition of knowledge and skills in the areas of counselling, instructing, caring, managing and communicating. Finally, continuous giving reinforces the importance of the balance in palliative care nursing between self-care needs and the complexities of death and dying.

The role of the physician

The physician on the team deals, in general, with complex symptom control problems as well as with issues related to the patients' and families' understanding of the diagnosis and prognosis. In addition, physicians on interdisciplinary teams have the responsibility to reflect and debate with other team members on their current medical management practices with regard to patients who are terminally ill. They need to clarify difficulties associated with end-of-life decision-making with the referring team, with the patients and their relatives. Furthermore, physicians have the responsibility of educating medical students, junior doctors and nurses on current practices in palliative care. They may also have a role in heightening the awareness of palliative care in other settings by presenting complex cases alongside other senior doctors and stimulating clinical research and publication of the team. Physicians working in palliative care must be competent in general medicine, have understanding of malignant disease and other diseases in the patient population and be familiar with hospice care. Besides this they will need the personal qualities of compassion, patience, maturity and confidence. The role of the physician may vary; some are attending physicians for hospice patients or for patients in the community or inpatient settings, while others enjoy a consultancy role.

The role of the social worker

The social worker may have an important role in interdisciplinary teams. He or she assesses and advises on the psychological, emotional and social problems of patients and their families.

The assessment of family attitudes and resources forms an integral part in the treatment plan for patients. The social worker uses individual, family or group work techniques in their assessment process. The social worker's contribution helps to highlight that every patient is part of a social system which influences how they deal with their illness (Dunlop & Hockley, 1998). Raymer (cited in Joisy, 1999) identified five specific goals that are consistent standards for social workers in palliative care:

(1) Enhancing the responsiveness of the environment
(2) Stimulating internal and psychological coping skills of the individual and his or her family
(3) Screening for psychopathology
(4) Enhancing the self-worth of the family system as well as the individual
(5) Providing specific symptom control.

Social workers also have a major role in organising care and placement for patients. Responsibility for co-ordinating bereavement follow-up work may also be given to the social worker of the team.

Besides having a clinical role, the social worker needs to be involved with the teaching activities of the team, especially in issues of communication and families. Because of their experience and knowledge social workers can also monitor feelings within the team.

The role of the clergy, chaplain or religious representative

The chaplain is often more a peripheral member than a core member of a palliative care team but has several important roles. The chaplain can help the team sort out spiritual and religious issues. He or she may act as a patient's advocate, taking into consideration the patient's and family's perspective. The spiritual member of the team may play an active role when it comes to ethical decisions and problems concerning end-of-life issues. Counselling patients and participating in bereavement follow-up are seen as core activities of the clergyman in the clinical environment. The clergy also has an important role in the basic religious requirements such as administering sacraments and praying for the dying. Finally, one should not underestimate the role of the clergy in educating the future physicians, nurses and other health professionals on issues dealing with death and dying.

One may argue that a team working together in collaborative palliative care offers the quality and depth of care that is not achievable by non-collaborative palliative care services or by independent practitioners. With this approach, emphasis is placed on the contribution of the interprofessional team to meet the present and anticipated needs of the patients and their families. By utilising a team approach, patient priorities are recognised, families are included in the decision-making process, suffering is minimised, individual team members are not over-burdened, and quality care is provided.

3.4   Conclusions

Palliative care can be provided by means of many different models of domiciliary and inpatient services. There is a tendency towards comprehensive programmes in which several disciplines and institutions work together in order to offer collaborative palliative care. Little is known about the content of the care that the services provide, the roles and tasks of the several disciplines, the needs for specialised skills and knowledge of the care providers, the organisation and financial resources of the care models or the barriers in implementing these models. More research in this area is warranted.

Chapter 4

Models of Palliative Care for Children

Huda Huijer Abu-Saad

4.1 Introduction

Palliative care can be defined as the active total care of children and their families by a multidisciplinary team when the child's disease is no longer responsive to curative treatment. Palliative care for children and young people with life-limiting conditions is an active and total approach to care, embracing physical, emotional, social and spiritual elements. It focuses on enhancement of quality of life for the child and support for the family and includes the management of distressing symptoms, provision of respite, and care through death and bereavement.

4.2 Life-limiting illnesses in palliative care

Fortunately, deaths in childhood for which palliative care may be applicable are rare. A report published by the Association for Children with Life-threatening or Terminal Conditions and their Families (ACT, 1997) and the Royal College of Pediatrics and Child Health offers the most up-to-date information on epidemiology:

- Annual mortality from life-limiting illnesses: 1 per 10 000 children aged 1–17 years
- Prevalence of life-limiting illnesses: 10 per 10 000 children aged 0–19 years
- In a health district of 250 000 people with a child population of about 50 000, in one year:
  - 5 children are likely to die from life-limiting illness – cancer (2), heart disease (1), and other (2)
  - 50 children are likely to have life-limiting illness, about half of whom will need palliative care at any time.

Palliative care in children may be needed for a wide range of diseases, which differ from adult diseases. The diagnosis will influence the type of care received. Palliative care may be needed from infancy and for many years for some children,

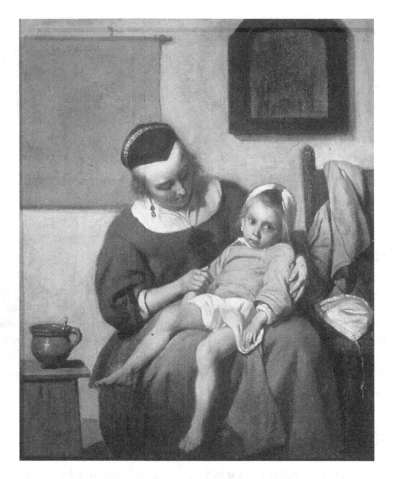

Fig. 4.1 Painting Mother and Child. (Reproduced with permission from the Rijksmuseum Amsterdam)

while others may not need it until they are older and for a short period of time (Goldman, 1998). In palliative care for children, life-limiting conditions are described as those for which there is no reasonable hope of cure and from which children will die. Many of these conditions cause progressive deterioration, rendering the child increasingly dependent on parents and carers. Four broad groups have been delineated (ACT, 1997):

(1) Life-threatening conditions for which curative treatment may be feasible but can fail. Palliative care may be necessary during periods of prognostic uncertainty and when treatment fails. Children in long-term remission or following successful curative treatment are not included. Examples: cancer and irreversible organ failures of heart, liver and kidney.

(2) Conditions where there may be long periods of intensive treatment aimed at prolonging life and allowing participation in normal childhood activities,

but premature death is still possible. Examples: cystic fibrosis and muscular dystrophy.

(3) Progressive conditions without curative treatment options, where treatment is exclusively palliative and may commonly extend over many years. Examples: Batten's disease and mucopolysaccharidosis.

(4) Conditions with severe neurological disability, which may cause weakness and susceptibility to health complications and may deteriorate unpredictably, but are not usually considered progressive. Examples: severe multiple disabilities such as following brain or spinal cord injuries, including some children with severe cerebral palsy.

Cancer is the most common cause of death in children between the ages of one and fourteen. Almost one-third of all children presenting with malignant disease will eventually die. A number of these children die suddenly and unexpectedly in hospital as a result of complications of their disease or its treatment. The majority of deaths in children are however predictable and are due to the malignancy itself. Under these circumstances the philosophy of care should shift from cure to care with emphasis on the physical, emotional, social and spiritual needs of the patients and family. According to Chambers and Oakhill (1995), children and their families prefer them to die at home in an environment in which they feel safe. Home-based pediatric palliative care services should in this respect focus on the close collaboration between a hospital-based palliative care team and the primary health care team. Care of the dying child should occur in the place of choice of child and family and should be provided by the expert health care professional known to them.

For most patients in palliative care and in particular for children there is usually a transitional period during which the focus of care shifts from treatments aimed at curing the disease or prolonging life towards palliative and supportive care. Figure 4.2 illustrates the time course of transition to palliative care that may vary depending on many factors such as the natural history of the underlying illness and the approach of health care professionals. Health care professionals and parents may have difficulty acknowledging the nature, severity and advanced stage of the child's illness and in accepting the reality of the situation. These and others have ramifications on the course of the transitional period.

4.3 Models of care

Services can be provided in many ways under the umbrella of paediatric (hospice) palliative care (Corr & Corr, 1985). Inpatient care can be provided in a variety of settings: a children's hospital, a paediatric medical centre, a general hospital or a designated hospice unit. Similarly home care can be provided in a variety of ways: community-based, hospital-based, or a combination of home-based co-ordinated by hospital and community staff. In addition a number of initiatives in different countries focus on the needs of the families during the terminal illness phase by providing respite care for the parents and siblings and after death by providing bereavement services for the whole family.

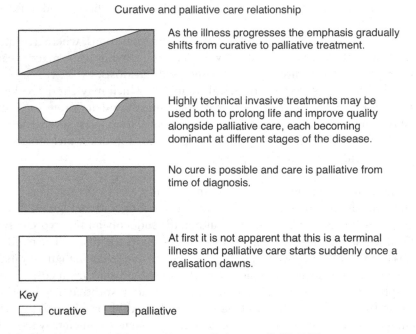

Curative and palliative care relationship

As the illness progresses the emphasis gradually shifts from curative to palliative treatment.

Highly technical invasive treatments may be used both to prolong life and improve quality alongside palliative care, each becoming dominant at different stages of the disease.

No cure is possible and care is palliative from time of diagnosis.

At first it is not apparent that this is a terminal illness and palliative care starts suddenly once a realisation dawns.

Key

☐ curative   ▨ palliative

Fig. 4.2   The time course of the transition to palliative care (ACT 1997).

The hospital can provide a sense of security for the child and family as well as the provision of continued care by health care professionals known to them. The disadvantages of hospital palliative care include the loss of control by the parents and taking care of their child in an environment that is institutional and rigid. In addition, for many families, a specialised hospital is usually far from home necessitating long commutes. Frequent visits may become difficult so that siblings and other members of the extended family may be excluded. A local hospital may be more convenient and conducive in providing care but may know the family less well and might lack confidence and experience in palliative care.

Being cared for in familiar surroundings is almost always the preference of the children. Family ties may be maintained, and life can go on as normally as possible with parents continuing to have control of their child's care. Heavy responsibility in this respect falls on the shoulders of the parents, as well as on the primary care provider, who feel in some respects ill-equipped to deal with a dying child. In order for home palliative care to be successful, support is inevitable. Many hospitals have developed as a result centrally-based home care teams that travel to the families' homes. In 1986 the provision of a hospital-based symptom care team at the Hospital for Sick Children, Great Ormond Street, resulted in a shift with regard to the place of death of a dying child. The percentage of families whose children died at home changed from 19% between 1978 and 1981 before the team began, to 75% between 1987 and 1989.

Hospices for children have found their developing role to be different from that of hospices for adults. Comparatively, few children with cancer have been admitted. Large numbers of children admitted to a hospice have long-term problems from metabolic and neurodegenerative diseases and many of the admissions are for respite care (Goldman, 1992). Hospices have played an important role for families with children with a long and slow disease trajectory and deterioration such as brain tumours. In addition, families with complex social and psychological circumstances making home care difficult have made use of hospice services.

The Paediatric Oncology Outreach Nurse Specialist (POONS) emerged in the 1980s as a nursing speciality area as a result of parental and nursing perceptions of gaps in services for families caring for a child with a malignant disease. The services were initially started to support families and carers through the ordeals of a terminal illness at home. They have been expanded since to include care through all stages of a child's illness. The POONS services have been largely funded through the Cancer and Leukemia in Childhood (CLIC) Charity and the Cancer Relief Macmillan Fund (CRMF) charity (Hunt, 1996). The principle aim of POONS is to bridge the gaps in services which can arise for children with malignant diseases and their families between primary, secondary and tertiary health care settings. Their aim is to provide links between this care triad in order to establish a seamless service throughout a child's illness. POONS act as a contact person for families in their homes during periods of treatment and thereafter. The type of support required of the nurses demands specialised skills and knowledge in helping the parents and the sick child deal with the terminal illness and adjust to another pattern of life. The support does extend beyond the death of the child and includes the bereavement period.

The paediatric oncology unit at the Royal Hospital for Sick Children in Bristol (Chambers & Oakhill, 1995) provides care for children diagnosed with cancer based on the principles of shared care. The care is provided by a consultant general paediatrician, a community oncology nurse, and an assistant specialist doctor who is responsible for the liaison with the tertiary centre specialists in Bristol. The nurse's role allows for liaisoning with the community services and patient's school, and for the continuing education of parents and patients concerning the nature of the disease and its treatment. Similarly Farrell and Sutherland (1998) describe a project where statutory and voluntary services collaborate to provide an effective range of services for children in palliative care. In particular, consideration is given to the experience of the children's hospice service and a paediatric oncology outreach service in providing palliative care to terminally ill children in the UK. The main aim of this project was to provide 'seamless care' and to ensure that partnership in care is achieved.

4.4   Palliative care at home

Martinson *et al.* (1977, 1978, 1986) and Martinson and Martinson (1983), based on pioneering work to determine the feasibility of home care as an alternative for the dying child, came up with a number of conditions which have to be met to make palliative home care for children possible:

- Cure-oriented treatment has to be discontinued
- The child desires to be at home
- The parents desire to have the child at home
- The parents believe they have the ability to care for the child at home
- The nurse and physician are available as consultants on a 24-hour basis.

In her studies Martinson describes how the roles of the physician, nurse and family are altered in home care. The family becomes the primary caregiver, the doctor acts as a consultant, and the nurse is seen as the facilitator of care.

Edwardson (1983), in a retrospective survey of parents who had cared for a dying child at home, found the prime influence on the choice for palliative care at home was the child's desire to be at home. The parents' ability to care for the child at home was ranked second. Other areas ranking high were the siblings' desires to have the terminally ill child at home. Carlson *et al.* (1985) found the availability of the nurse on a 24-hour basis to positively influence the decision for home care. Kohler and Radford (1985), based on their studies for home care, cited two major reasons for home care: the child's desires and keeping the family together. Walsh (1987) emphasised the cultural differences that could influence the choice for home care versus hospital care. She made reference to the Japanese culture that would more likely choose hospital care because of their beliefs of keeping spirits of death away from home. Bluebond-Langer (1978), based on observations of children with terminal cancer, reported on the other hand the existence of fear among children about being treated at home. These children were afraid that they would not receive adequate care at home. In some situations this might be a valid concern and consequently deserves further investigation before developing palliative care services for children.

Lauer *et al.* (1986), in a study looking at prevalence, utilisation and efficacy of home care services for children in the USA, surveyed 85 institutions in 45 states. Of these institutions, 86% offered home care services, of which 44% were self-administered while the remainder relied on community-based resources. The programmes operating from institutions had a larger proportion of families using them, reported a lower hospital death rate, and provided more structured visits and as a result less crisis intervention. The community agencies encountered a number of problems, including inexperience in paediatric care, inadequate symptom recognition and management, and reluctance of families to work with unfamiliar health professionals.

Duffy *et al.* (1990) in an evaluation study of palliative care services in Toronto, Canada, reported that the institution of a home care programme for children with central nervous system tumours had resulted in more deaths at home and fewer total number of hospitalisation days in the terminal phase of their illness. In addition, the parents were more satisfied with the care provided and in particular there was satisfaction at being able to care for their child at home with access to specialist care. The main characteristics of this programme were the presence of a nurse co-ordinator with three palliative care nurses and a clinical pharmacist. The team worked closely with the primary care physician and community services. Similarly, an article describing a home-based palliative care service developed at the Children's Hospital in Philadelphia, emphasised the notion of team work between parents, a palliative care physician, home care nurses, social workers and bereavement specialists.

In a retrospective chart review conducted by Kopecky *et al.* (1997), the utilisation of the above-mentioned Toronto home-based palliative care programme for children was studied. The study included 126 children admitted between 1986 and 1994 to the Hospital for Sick Children in Toronto with malignant and non-malignant diseases. Of the 93 patients who died, 53% died at home, 18% died in community hospitals, and 29% died in a tertiary care facility. Analgesic medications were administered to 54% of the patients, and 56% of these required opioid analgesia for pain and symptom control. The home-based palliative care programme for children was found to be feasible, providing another option for some terminally ill children and their parents.

Collins *et al.* (1998), in a study conducted in Australia on 'home care for the dying child; a parent's perception', cited a number of benefits of home care versus hospital care. Greater freedom, more privacy, and less disruption of family life were cited often by the parents in the study. In addition emphasis was placed on the experience of caring for one's child in a familiar environment, which was seen and valued by all parents as a positive experience.

Despite these experiences many families expressed a number of fears and concerns with regard to the symptomatic care of their child and the type of support they received. A number of families experienced difficulties with regard to hospital readmission of their child during palliative care when pain, discomfort and distress at home were no longer manageable. Many parents experienced the night to be the most difficult. Certainly support at night was less available and parents developed chronic fatigue by taking shifts and in some cases maintaining a vigil at the bedside. Feelings of isolation and loneliness surfaced often.

This study also showed that the longer the child's illness the more likely the parent was to adjust to the illness and put the cancer experience in perspective. Conversely, the shorter the duration, the less likely that parents would adjust successfully. The study concluded with a number of recommendations for effective support of parents as caregivers of the child dying at home:

- Allow parents to choose between hospital-based or home-based palliative care, with the option to switch if need arises
- Ensure availability of professional support 24 hours a day, seven days a week
- Provide parents with adequate information on drug treatment and what to expect
- Provide assistance with routine home duties
- Provide relief at night to ensure adequate sleep
- Provide respite care
- Avoid administrative delays when readmission to hospital is required
- Provide family doctors and community nurses with additional information.

In a study addressing the needs of parents of pediatric oncology patients during the palliative care phase, James & Johnson (1997) identified three categories of needs:

- The need to have the child recognised as special while retaining as much normality as possible within the child's and family's lives
- The need for caring and connectedness with health care professionals
- The need to retain responsibility of parenting their dying child.

Lack of information was an issue for parents. Communication between parent and health professionals of sufficient and timely information may enhance feelings of usefulness by inherently increasing parents' ability to care for their child at home. The identified needs can be seen as illustrations of parents struggling during a time of anguish for the whole family. The study showed as well that against all odds, the parents wanted to preserve some normality for the child, themselves and other family members and they had tremendous needs for care and support from the health care professionals during this time.

In an exploratory, descriptive study of the experiences in five different countries of mothers whose child died of cancer, Davies *et al.* (1998) found no culturally related differences. The mothers' recall of the experiences was found to be more similar than different. All mothers reacted with shock, disbelief, fear, sadness and anger to the news of their children's diagnoses. Mothers preferred to care for their children at home during the final phase of the illness. They all agreed that home provided a happier and more 'normal' environment for the children. They felt comfortable managing care at home, as long as they could depend on professional caregivers who could offer assistance when needed. Perceived uncontrolled symptoms were seen as reasons to admit the child to the hospital. The children themselves preferred the comfort, security and familiarity of their own homes. Fathers were also involved in the care of the terminally ill child at home. Siblings on the other hand were found to be minimally involved. This was found to be of concern, because surviving siblings are particularly vulnerable and should not be forgotten. This study is of particular relevance to the field of cross-cultural palliative care research and practice. It has provided us with valuable information on mothers' perceptions and preferences for the place of death of their child. The preference for palliative care at home was not dependent on the differences in available services in the different countries.

Dangel *et al.* (2000) using survey methods evaluated the quality of the Warsaw pediatric hospice home care programme in Poland. A total of 136 parents received questionnaires, of which 80 were returned. Results showed that the majority of the caregivers preferred home over hospital care. Keeping the family together and the preference of the child to be at home were cited as important factors in their decision. At home, feelings of helplessness and fear were most common and most difficult to handle among caregivers. The majority of the parents were not able to speak honestly with their children about their impending death. Most of the children, however, died peacefully at home and did not suffer. Satisfaction with the hospice home care programme was high. Results obtained from this study are seen as useful in improving the quality of servive delivery in Poland and in impacting on health care policy in this area.

In some situations home-based palliative care might not be easy; it demands a great deal of support from the community, hospital and medical and nursing services. In addition, the parents may not have the physical and emotional resources to deal with it. Although in most cases these practical problems can be overcome by mobilising the right resources, one needs to listen to assess the needs and capabilities of the parents before a decision regarding palliative care is made. In some cases an alternative to home or hospital-based palliative care may be a hospice. There are at the moment many children's hospices in the UK and in the USA. The foremost of these is Helen House in Oxford (Fig. 4.3), which was the first hospice in the world established to look after dying children.

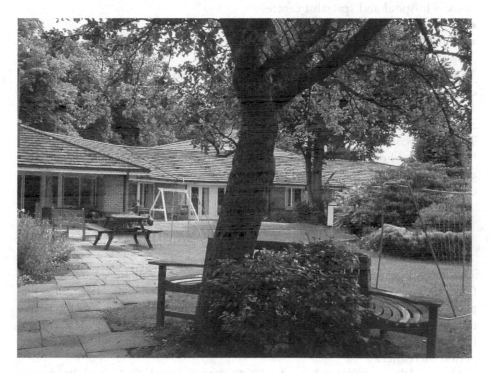

Fig. 4.3   Helen House Hospice for Children

Looking at cost issues, Martinson *et al.* (1977) reported practical economic benefits of home care compared to hospital care. Moldow *et al.* (1982) found the costs for hospital care to range from 20%–200% more than home care of the child with terminal cancer. The wide variation was related to whether the home care was purely an alternative to hospital care or whether it represented a broader concept of care, including times the child needed hospitalisation. Other authors emphasise that the value of home care is related to the psychological benefits to the patients and their families.

Estimating the cost of palliative care remains complicated. Newer programmes frequently underestimate the total costs due to inconsistencies in analysing or acknowledging indirect expenses. Incidental expenses for non-medical purchases and supplies incurred in caring for the child at home can also be substantial for some families. The cost of lost wages by some caregivers can constitute a significant fraction of costs incurred by the family. These types of financial stressors need to be identified and adequately assessed when cost comparisons are made.

Goldman (1996) lists a number of aspects that need to be included in a home palliative care programme:

- 24-hour access to expertise in paediatric and family care
- 24-hour access to expertise in paediatric palliative care
- A key worker to co-ordinate the care between family, carers in the community, local hospital and specialist centres
- Respite care facilities
- Immediate access to hospital if needed.

This model could be used to develop more comprehensive systems of care for children dying from diseases other than cancer. Goldman *et al.* (1990) in their article on models of palliative care in children concluded that children who were receiving potentially curative treatments were more likely to die in the hospital. This was in contrast with children receiving palliative treatments who were more likely to die at home or in a hospice. The choice depended on the condition of the child, the available resources and the confidence of the parents in caring for the ill child at home.

4.5   Development of multidisciplinary guidelines

The development of guidelines is an essential part of palliative care services. Guidelines refer to two periods in the final phase of life of a child. The first is the period when the treatment is judged to be no longer effective and a decision needs to be made to move from curative to palliative care. The second is the period from the beginning of palliative care to the death of the child and the bereavement period thereafter.

The guidelines developed by the SIOP (International Society of Paediatric Oncology) working committee on psychosocial oncology (Masera *et al.*, 1999) emphasise the right of the terminally ill child to die without unnecessary pain, fear or anxiety and how essential it is that he or she receives adequate medical, spiritual and psychosocial support. It is just as important that the child at no point in the disease trajectory feels abandoned either by the health professionals, the health centre or by his/her family. Palliative care in the terminal phase should be tailored to the needs and desires of the child and the family, with the goal of providing the best possible quality of life for the days that remain. Truly essential are absolute love, commitment and understanding from all involved. How the child's death is handled will have a tremendous influence on the survivors, mainly the family, siblings and other close family, and will profoundly affect their lives.

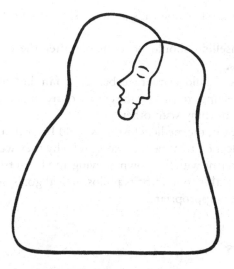

Fig. 4.4   Fusion in care (Courtesy of Simon Andras, Budapest)

Guidelines for the transition from the curative to the palliative phase (Masera et al. 1999)

- The centre should develop a uniform philosophy on key issues such as pain management, communication and support
- The parents, alongside the health care team, should be involved in the decision-making process from the beginning of treatment and throughout the course of the disease. The child, depending on age and development, should also be involved.
- Parents' wishes may not always be the best for the child. Members of the health care team should take time to understand and discuss unrealistic wishes such as pursuing an unrealistic possibility for cure or stopping curative treatment prematurely. By doing so, inevitably painful conflicts can be overcome.
- The continuation of curative treatment beyond the point when cure is no longer possible, should be avoided (the so-called 'ruthless obstinacy' treatment).

Guidelines during palliative care and thereafter (Masera et al. 1999)

- The decision needs to be made by the caring team. Physical pain control must be carried out with professional competence along with the management of all other emerging symptoms such as vomiting, constipation and bladder control.
- Children wishing to stay at home should be allowed to do so. Provision should be made for professional support at home.
- Parents and health care teams should stay attuned to the child in the terminal phase and should reflect on what the child communicates.

- Follow-up visits and telephone calls at home should be offered by the physician.
- Bereavement counselling should be available after the child's death to the family and siblings.
- Health care teams should encourage bereaved families to initiate self-help groups to discuss feelings regarding the course of treatment and palliation and for sharing their mourning with others.
- After the child's death, the medical history should be evaluated by the team. It is important to reflect on treatment choices and why they were made. This will help staff come to terms with their own grieving and learn from the experience.
- The team should be able to modify its philosophical goals and reset directions and guidelines when appropriate.

4.6   Conclusions

In summary, for home-based paediatric palliative care to be effective, it is essential that cure-oriented treatment be discontinued and that there is an evident desire from the child and the parents to be at home. In addition, the parents need to have the confidence and ability to take care of a terminally ill child at home. This can, however, be acquired through adequate training and support. Furthermore, the family should have access to 24-hour medical and nursing services and support. Finally, the success of any programme is dependent on the knowledge and skills of the health professionals involved. Additional training of physicians, nurses and other health professionals involved in the care of the terminally ill child is highly warranted.

Chapter 5
Evaluation of Palliative Care

Huda Huijer Abu-Saad

5.1 Introduction

Palliative care is a rapidly expanding speciality area in health care. It plays an important role in providing services to enable terminally ill patients and their families to deal effectively with symptom control and management and to improve quality of life. The effectiveness of palliative care services has recently received a great deal of attention. Effectiveness in palliative care is judged in terms of the quality of life of patient and family, the adequacy of symptom control, and the satisfaction of the patient and family with the care received. Besides effectiveness, efficiency plays an important role in evaluating palliative care services. Issues relating to quality of care with cost-effectiveness are of particular interest here. Although randomised controlled trials are considered the gold standard in evaluating effectiveness in this field, they are still rare. Methodological and ethical issues in conducting studies with this patient group have contributed to this difficulty.

This chapter reviews studies conducted in this area, which are summarised in Table 5.1. A total number of 48 studies were identified, including randomised controlled trials, and comparative and observational studies. In order to provide as complete a picture as possible on the use of palliative care services, survey studies denoting the state of the art in the different countries are also included.

5.2 Population-based studies

In a population-based study conducted in Italy on all cancer deaths between 1986 and 1990, Constantini *et al.* (1993) found that the percentage of home deaths increased over that period, with twice as many among palliative home care users compared with non-users. Palliative home care users were found in general to be younger, married, and more highly educated. The probability of home death was found to increase with increasing age and education level, and was higher in females and in married patients. The provision of palliative home care was the strongest predictor of home death.

De Conno *et al.* (1996), in a prospective evaluation study of the home care programme provided for patients with advanced cancer in Milan, found that

86% of the patients died at home and 14% in hospital. The presence of a high degree of family support was associated with home death. The quality of pain control was found to be improved in patients dying at home, while physical debility and cognitive functioning were found to worsen throughout the home care duration. Psychological distress such as anxiety and depression was high at the end of life and was not affected by treatment.

In a survey by Voltz *et al.* (1997), terminally ill patients in the USA, Germany and Japan were interviewed by their health care providers. In the USA there was a substantial difference in the admission of non-cancer patients compared with Germany and Japan. Considering the informed consent procedure, in the USA and Germany the patients were well informed, but in Japan only about 60% of the patients knew the diagnosis, the nature of the disease process and their medical condition at the time of their admission. In Japan, explicit oral consent was mostly obtained from the families.

5.3   Effectiveness studies

In a study designed to evaluate the effects of a hospice consultation team, Abrahm *et al.* (1996) interviewed 75 cancer patients. Results showed that the consultation team led to improvement in identification and management of patient problems, better relief of pain, and more attention to the psychosocial and spiritual problems of patients. In a similar study Addington-Hall *et al.* (1992) measured the effects of co-ordinating services on symptom control, satisfaction and costs. Results showed improvement in costs and slightly better symptom control, but no difference in satisfaction. Ballinx (1995) in a study conducted in Belgium found an improvement in STAS (Support Team Assessment Schedule) scores in favour of the palliative care support team. Similarly, Higginson & Hearn (1997) and Higginson *et al.* (1990, 1992) found support teams to be effective in reducing symptoms and improving satisfaction of cancer patients and families.

Edmonds *et al.* (1998), using an expanded STAS, studied symptom prevalence and outcome among inpatients and outpatients referred to a multiprofessional hospital palliative care team. E-STAS forms were completed on referral and twice weekly thereafter. Of the symptoms assessed on referral the most common were psychological distress (93%), anorexia (73%), pain (59%), mouth discomfort (59%), depression (40%), constipation (36%), breathlessness (32%), nausea (24%) and vomiting (13%). Results showed statistically significant improvements from first to last assessments in all symptoms except depression. Patient-generated and proxy-generated scores were found to be highly correlated with proxies rating patients as slightly more impaired than patients themselves.

Butters *et al.* (1992, 1993) evaluated the effects of community palliative care teams by AIDS patients. Results showed an improvement in symptom control and in particular pain and anxiety, and more satisfaction with care. Ellershaw (1995) found in addition palliative care teams to be more effective in reducing pain, nausea and constipation and in improving nutritional support of patients with terminal cancer. More satisfaction with care and lower costs were also found by

Campbell (1996) when evaluating the effectiveness of supportive palliative care teams as seen by families of terminally ill patients. Cartwright and Seale (1990) also used the experiences of relatives of patients who died of cancer to evaluate palliative care. Their results showed better quality of care at time of death, more satisfaction with care and better care provided by nurses at home.

In a published review article Hearn and Higginson (1998) studied the effectiveness of palliative care teams. The objective of the study was to determine whether teams providing specialist palliative care do improve the health outcomes of patients with terminal cancer and their carers when compared with conventional services. Outcomes used in this systematic review included different aspects of symptom control, patient and family or carer satisfaction, health care utilisation, cost, place of death, psychosocial indices and quality of life. Based on a thorough search of the literature using different databases and personal contacts with authors, and utilising a self-developed evaluation index, 18 relevant articles were identified including five randomised control trials. Results showed improved outcomes in specialist teams when compared with conventional care. There was evidence of increased satisfaction of patients and carers, better symptom control, reduction in hospital days, reduction in costs, more time spent at home by patients, and increased likelihood of patients dying where they wished. The authors concluded that multiprofessional approaches to palliative care using a specialist team do have an impact on the quality of care delivered and on reducing the overall costs.

Greer *et al.* (1986), in a quasi-experimental study comparing home and hospital-based hospice care with conventional care, found pain and symptom control and perceived burden and emotional stress to be improved in hospice care. Costs of hospice care were found to be lower than conventional care. No difference in patient satisfaction with care was found. In a prospective study comparing hospital care with hospice care, Hinton (1979) found that hospice patients scored better on depression, anxiety and anger; they were better aware of their diagnosis; and they were more satisfied with the care they received. In a more recent study to evaluate palliative home care services, Hinton (1996) found an improvement in symptom management which was related to the frequent individual care provided by palliative home care nurses.

Hughes *et al.* (1992) in a randomised controlled trial studied the effects of a hospital-based home care programme for terminally ill patients. Results showed an improvement in satisfaction with care, a reduction in total hospital days, and lower costs. Similarly in a randomised controlled trial, Kane *et al.* (1984, 1985ab, 1986) studied the effects of hospice care for cancer patients. Results showed an improvement in satisfaction with interpersonal care and in the degree of involvement in care. No differences were found, however, in pain control and in reducing anxiety and depression. McWhinney *et al.* (1994), using a randomised controlled design to evaluate the effectiveness of a palliative home care, also found no difference in symptom control and other measures.

Vinciguerra *et al.* (1986) studied the effectiveness of palliative care at home compared with hospital care. Results showed improved survival and decreased use of analgesics for home care patients compared with hospital care patients. A non-randomised study of Tsainandouraki *et al.*(1992), however, showed that patients who were treated in the home care programme had poor survival compared to those treated at the hospital over a 60-month period. Due to flaws in study design, results of this study cannot be regarded as conclusive. They do indicate, however, that hospitalisation may have a substantial impact on survival in terminally ill patients. In a study of Tamarin *et al.* (1992), hospital care was compared with home palliative care. Results showed an increase in well being and an estimated annual saving of 35% in home care compared with hospital care. Peruselli *et al.* (1997), in a more recent prospective study evaluating the effects of palliative home care, also found home care to be more effective in mitigating pain and other symptoms and in reducing psychological distress.

In a study evaluating the effectiveness of home care when compared to hospital care, Ventafridda *et al.* (1989) found home care to be more effective in improving performance status and quality of life and in reducing costs. No differences were found, however, in reducing pain and other symptoms. In comparing the quality of life of cancer patients dying on palliative care units and in hospitals, Viney *et al.* (1994) found improvement in expressed good feelings, and less expressed anger and anxiety. No differences, however, were found in quality of life between the two groups. Finally, in a study of Dessloch *et al.* (1992), perceptions from terminally ill patients in hospitals were compared with terminally ill patients at home. The variable 'positivism perceived from the environment' like 'a good atmosphere at home' and 'feelings of control' were experienced more at home. 'Satisfaction with medical and nursing care' was perceived to be equally good at home and in the hospital.

5.4   Cost-effectiveness studies

Bierenbaum & Kidder (1984) found a difference in costs when comparing hospital-based hospice care with home-based hospice care regardless of length of stay. In a retrospective study Bierenbaum (1992) compared in addition hospital and home care costs of terminal care in childhood cancer. Overall home care was found to be less expensive than hospital terminal care, except when non-health care and indirect care costs were considered. Using hospital insurance claims, Brooks & Smyth Staruch (1984) compared hospice home care with conventional care. The effects of care cost savings to third party insurers were examined when home care visits were substituted for hospital inpatient days. The cost savings were substantial showing a 50% decrease in hospital use and a tenfold increase in home care visits.

A prospective study with terminal AIDS patients (Tamarin *et al.* 1992), where home care was compared to hospital care, showed cost savings when palliative care was provided at home. Efficiency of the care team's access to patients, family support, and the resultant reduction of patient admission accounted for these results. Furthermore, Mor *et al.* (1985) and Greer *et al.* (1986) compared home hospice care and hospital hospice care costs with conventional care costs and found a difference in costs in favour of home hospice care. Contrary to the results mentioned above, Gray & Elder (1987) found no significant differences in costs when the total costs of hospice home care and conventional terminal care during the last 90 days of life were compared.

Hill & Oliver (1984, 1989), in evaluating costs of inpatient hospice care, found costs of inpatient hospice care to depend on the number of beds in hospice units. Units with a lower number of beds have higher costs per bed per week. Bly & Kissinck (1994) compared hospice home care given to regular hospice patients with this type of care given to 'living alone patients' (LAPs) at home. Although the hospice care providers were able to provide care safely while letting the LAPs die at home, the costs in caring for LAPs tended to be higher than those for regular hospice patients. Carlson *et al.* (1988) evaluated the effects of comprehensive supportive palliative care teams on cost savings and found the teams to be effective in reducing hospital stays, resulting in fewer services provided by the hospital. Field *et al.* (1996) found similar results. In a randomised controlled trial, Raftery *et al.* (1996) tested the effectiveness of a co-ordinated service for terminally ill cancer patients. The service was found to be cost-effective when compared with standard services, due to achieving the same outcomes at lower service use.

Axelsson and Christensen (1998) compared the financial benefits of a hospital-based palliative support service with a matched historical control group and a group of contemporary reference patients. Results of this evaluation study showed that patients in the study group had shorter terminal admissions, a greater proportion of days at home during the enrolment period, and more days at home during the last two months of life compared with the control group. The cost of running this service corresponded to six institutional days per patient and was found to be self-financing. The provision of appropriate support to domiciliary care allows terminally ill patients to spend more time at home and gives them a realistic choice as to where they want to end their lives. This will result in decreasing medical costs to society, which is by itself a major reward, according to the authors. With regard to the unpaid workload borne by the family members and friends, no differences were found between the study group and the reference group concerning the number of family members' days off work needed to support the patient at home.

Table 5.1 Effectiveness of palliative care models

Author and country	Purpose of the study	Patient population	Study design	Major outcomes	Major results
Abrahm *et al.* (1996) USA	To evaluate the effects of a hospice consultation team	75 cancer patients	Evaluation study	Pain Medical/nursing health care problems	Improvement in identification and management of patient problems Better relief of pain More attention to psychosocial and spiritual problems
Addington-Hall *et al.* (1992) UK	To measure the effects on terminally ill cancer patients and their families of co-ordinating the services and to compare cost effectiveness of the service	203 cancer patients with a prognosis of one year	Randomised controlled trial	Symptom control ADL Satisfaction Hospital anxiety and depression scale (HADS) QoL Carers' experience and satisfaction Depression and anxiety scale for carers Costs	Improvement in: fewer days in hospital fewer home visits lower costs fewer anger feelings No difference in: satisfaction with services unmet needs
Axelsson & Christensen (1998) Sweden	Financial assessment of a hospital-based palliative support service compared to matched historical control group and contemporary reference group	Cancer patients	Quasi-experimental design	Total institutional days Admissions last 6 months Days spent at home Ratio days spent at home to inclusion days Days at home last 6 months of life	Shorter terminal admissions Greater proportion of days at home during enrolment period More days at home last 6 months of life Service self-financing

	Aim	Sample	Evaluation study	Measures	Results
Ballinx (1995) Belgium	To evaluate the effects of a palliative care support team	109 patients		Support team assessment schedule (STAS)	Improvement in STAS scores
Bierenbaum & Kidder (1984) USA	To compare home care with conventional hospital care	11 hospital-based hospices 14 home-based hospices	Survey	Costs	Hospital-based hospice costs per day are 44% higher than home care hospice costs per day Per patient hospice costs are 20% higher in hospital than at home
Bierenbaum (1992) USA	Home care compared with conventional hospital care	8 hospital care patients (children) 11 home care patients (children)	Retrospective survey (interviews)	Direct health care costs (out/inpatient/home care) Indirect costs (e.g. income loss/counselling/donated equipment) Direct non-health care costs (e.g. lifestyle alterations/additional family expenses)	Total costs are lower in home care than in hospital care Non-health care costs and indirect costs at home are higher than in hospital
Bly & Kissinck (1994) USA	To evaluate hospice home care	34 living alone patients (LAPs) 105 hospice patients	Programme evaluation	Total costs: routine home care case management respite care inpatient care	LAPs enabled to die at home Staff provided safety and security LAPs required more supportive services and have higher patient costs than regular hospice patients

Table 5.1 Contd.

Author and country	Purpose of the study	Patient population	Study design	Major outcomes	Major results
Brooks & Smyth Staruch (1984) USA	To compare home hospice care with hospital hospice care	152 hospice patients 1397 conventional patients	Retrospective population-based survey	Hospital insurance claims	Decrease in hospital use Increase in home care visits Increased savings
Butters et al. (1992, 1993) UK	To evaluate the effects of community palliative care teams	140 AIDS patients 19 AIDS patients	Effect and process evaluation	Support team assessment schedule (STAS) Satisfaction	Less pain and other physical complaints Less anxiety More satisfaction with care
Campbell (1996) USA	To evaluate the effect of a supportive palliative care team	35 family members of terminal patients and their professional carers	Evaluation study	Satisfaction with care	Major results after referral to team: shorter hospital stay less curative interventions lower costs more satisfaction
Carlson et al. (1988) USA	To evaluate the effects of a comprehensive supportive palliative care	99 patients	Retrospective study	Health services utilisation	Shorter hospital stays Fewer services provided by hospital
Cartwright & Seale (1990) UK	To compare the experience of hospice cancer patients with other cancer patients	171 relatives of patients who died from cancer	800 registered deaths selected from 10 randomly chosen areas of England stratified by availability of hospice services	Questionnaire administered by interviewers on symptoms, services, information about medical procedures, involvement of family and friends in care	Improvement in: provision and frequency of visits by a nurse at home time spent talking rating of nursing care control of pain quality of care at time of death visit by a nurse after death

Study	Aim	Sample	Design	Variables	Results
Dessloch *et al.* (1992) Germany	To compare hospital to home hospice care	41 patients	Interviews	Burden of illness Social support Coping Feelings of control Satisfaction with medical and nursing care Physical stability	No significant differences were found Satisfaction perceived as good in both home and hospital
Edmonds *et al.* (1998) UK	To determine symptom prevalence and outcome for inpatients and outpatients referred to hospital palliative care team	352 cancer patients	Programme evaluation Forms completed at referral and twice weekly thereafter	Expanded STAS Psychological distress Anorexia Pain Mouth discomfort Depression Constipation Breathlessness Nausea Vomiting	Statistically significant improvements between first and last assessment in all symptoms except depression
Ellershaw (1995) UK	To evaluate the effects of an advisory palliative care team	125 cancer patients	Evaluation study	Palliative care assessment Pain and symptom management	Less pain, nausea, sedation and constipation Better nutritional support
Field *et al.* (1996) USA	To evaluate the effects of a comprehensive palliative care support team	40 terminal patients	Retrospective evaluation study	Mortality Health services utilisation	Shorter hospital stays Less use of hospital resources and curative interventions

Table 5.1 Contd.

Author and country	Purpose of the study	Patient population	Study design	Major outcomes	Major results
Gray & Elder (1987) Australia	To compare hospice home care with conventional care	98 patients who died in hospice service 98 patients who died in conventional terminal care	Retrospective case-control	Bed day costs Medical and nursing services Procedures and investigation	No significant differences in costs Bed day costs account for biggest part of total costs
Greer et al. (1986) USA	To compare home and hospital hospice care with conventional care	88 home care patients 624 hospital-based hospice patients 297 conventional care patients	Quasi-experimental	Costs Quality of life Pain and symptom management Satisfaction with care Perceived anxiety Perceived burden Morbidity	Costs of hospital care less than conventional care No difference in QoL Pain and symptom control improved in hospice care No difference in satisfaction with care and perceived anxiety Perceived burden and emotional stress less in hospice care No difference in morbidity
Hatcliff et al. (1996) UK	To evaluate home care services	148 district nurses	Survey	Experience in caring Educational needs Views of palliative care team	69% cared for dying patients over past 12 months Further education needed in pain and symptom management and in bereavement care Satisfied with team work Improvement in communication needed

Study	Aim	Sample	Study type	Measures	Results
Higginson et al. (1990) UK	To investigate the needs, views and problems of terminally ill cancer patients	65 cancer patients with family member/carer Mean age 66	Prospective study of patients receiving care from two multiprofessional support teams	Interview on current problems Rating on care Ratings on health services by MDs, RNs, GPs and support team staff	Excellent ratings for MDs, RNs, and GPs Negative ratings on hospital services communication, GPs' attitudes
Higginson et al. (1992) UK	Assess effectiveness of two support teams	227 in care for two or more weeks Mean age 67	Prospective observational	Support team assessment schedule (STAS)	Proportion of patients with severe problems reduced Scores on 15 out of 17 items improved
Higginson & Hearn (1997) Ireland and UK	To evaluate the effectiveness of hospital palliative care teams	695 cancer patients	Evaluation study	Support team assessment schedule (STAS)	Pain significantly less
Hill & Oliver (1984, 1989) UK	To evaluate inpatient hospice units	20 hospices (1984) 40 hospices (1989)	Survey	Inpatient care costs	Fall in costs with increasing bed numbers
Hinton (1979) UK	Compare care in hospital and hospice	80 cancer patients with <3 months prognosis Mean age 58.2	Prospective comparison study	Interviews provide visual analogue scale ratings on emotional state, attitude to illness, opinions on care	Hospice patients scored better on depression, anxiety and anger, were better aware of diagnosis, and expressed better praise. No difference in opinion on medical treatment

Table 5.1 Contd.

Author and country	Purpose of the study	Patient population	Study design	Major outcomes	Major results
Hinton (1996) UK	To evaluate home care services	77 patients	Prospective randomised survey	Contacts between professional carers and patients Types of care Pattern of care in relation to problem Service changes	Home care/community nurses most frequently contact patients Maintaining contact, giving explanations and support, physical treatment, practical nursing Help succeeded for nausea/vomiting, breathlessness, depression or constipation Weakness and pain Strengthening linkage between nurses and patients and improvement of day care services led to rise in patients dying at home

Author	Aim	Sample	Design	Measures	Results
Hughes *et al.* (1992) USA	To study the effect of a hospital-based home care programme on terminally ill patients and caregivers	171 terminally ill male patients with prognosis <6 months	Randomised controlled trial	Barthel's self-care index Satisfaction with care Health care utilisation	Improvement in: satisfaction with care reduction in total hospital days number of outpatient visits fewer days spent in hospital lower costs No difference in: percentage readmitted to hospital place of death
Jones 1993, Jones *et al.* (1993) UK	To identify levels of support and identify deficiencies of care	207 carers of patients who died at home Mean age 60	Observational with retrospective data collection by interview	Semi-structured interviews on sources of support, satisfaction and coping in the four weeks before death	Services judged as excellent Health care professionals had to listen and were caring GPs fared worst overall, difficulty getting urgent help
Kane *et al.* (1984, 1985a,b, 1986) USA	To assess the effect of hospice care on the emotional status of patients and caregivers	247 cancer patients with a prognosis of two weeks to six months	Randomised controlled trial	McGill pain questionnaire Symptom scale Anxiety scale Anger	Improvement in: satisfaction with interpersonal care Involvement in care No difference in: pain control satisfaction symptoms, anxiety, depression

Table 5.1   Contd.

Author and country	Purpose of the study	Patient population	Study design	Major outcomes	Major results
King et al. (1993) Scotland	To evaluate hospice services	11 hospices	Survey	Volunteer input Admissions Services Staffing Financial statement Crude average cost per case	No conclusions can be drawn Policies vary between hospices with regard to finance
Lunt & Neale (1987) UK	To compare the care goals of doctors and nurses working in hospices and general hospitals	86 patients recruited at random All nurses and doctors involved with patients	Quasi-experimental prospective study	Interviews with doctors and nurses based on Kiresuk's goal attainment scaling technique Interviews with patients	Differences between hospital and hospice Hospice MDs set more rehabilitation goals Hospice MDs set more goals for patients' physical comfort and emotional state Difference between staff and patients More concerns about emotional states by hospice Patients had concerns which they kept private; staff did not know about

Author	Aim	Sample	Design	Measures	Results
McCusker & Stoddard (1987) USA	To test the hypothesis that an expanded home care programme for the terminally ill would reduce hospitalisation and costs	1874 decedents who made claims during last six months of life	Quasi-experimental time series design	Acute hospital claims Long-term facility claims Home care claims	Greater savings among home users achieved by reduction in hospital days and reduction in mean daily cost of hospitalisation
McWhinney et al. (1994) Canada	To evaluate a home care team based on an inpatient unit	146 adult patients at home with a prognosis of two months	Randomised controlled trial Follow-up at one and two months	McGill Pain Questionnaire Nausea questionnaire	No difference in any measures between groups at one month
Mor et al. (1985) USA	To compare hospice care with hospital care	25 hospices 14 conventional oncology care settings	NHS survey	Inpatient costs Ancillary costs (Non) hospice home services costs	Costs less in hospice care compared to conventional care
Mor et al. (1988a,b) USA	To evaluate inpatient and home care hospice programmes against conventional care	1754 hospice and non-hospice patients	Prospective study of patients and carers attending hospice and 14 conventional care services	Pattern of care and treatments given Patient outcomes Overall quality of life Family outcomes Anxiety and burden, distress and morbidity Health care utilisation and costs	Improvement in: pain control and analgesic prescription less intensive interventions higher hours of direct care more likely to die at home lower costs No difference in: quality of life patient satisfaction family outcomes after death

Table 5.1 Contd.

Author and country	Purpose of the study	Patient population	Study design	Major outcomes	Major results
Parkes (1979, 1984) UK	To evaluate hospice with hospital care	34 patients and 34 matched controls	Retrospective analysis of views of bereaved spouses 13 months after death	Semi-structured interviews on effects of service on the patients' physical and psychosocial well being and on spouses	Improvement in severity of patient's pain, mobility Spouses spent more time with patient, were less worried
Parkes (1980, 1985) UK	To evaluate hospice advisory domiciliary service	51 patients and 51 matched controls who died of cancer	Retrospective analysis of views of bereaved spouses 13 months after death	Views of home care services, services required, communication, symptoms, patient contentment, time spent at home and readmission	Time in hospital reduced Reduction in costs No difference in symptoms Greater tension and anxiety when patient at home
Peruselli *et al.* (1997) Italy	To evaluate outcomes of palliative home care	106 advanced cancer patients	Prospective	Katz activity of daily living (ADL) Symptom distress scale	Palliative home care effective in mitigating pain Palliative home care in part effective in stimulating appetite, curbing nausea and controlling psychological distress

Author (Year) Country	Aim	Sample	Design	Measures	Results
Raftery *et al.* (1996) UK	To compare the cost-effectiveness of a co-ordination service with standard services for terminally ill cancer patients	167 cancer patients: 86 in co-ordination group and 81 in control group	Randomised controlled trial	Use of health and palliative care services. Differential costs to patients and carers	Lower mean total costs in co-ordination group. Mean cost per co-ordinated patient half that of control patient
Tierney *et al.* (1994) UK	To compare care provided in hospices	1 independent hospice 1 NHS hospice	In-depth case study	Costs per patient: direct and indirect costs fixed overhead costs	No substantial cost differences between two hospices
Tamarin (1992) Italy	To compare home care with hospital care	10 home care patients 32 hospital care patients	6-months prospective study	Quality of life and direct costs incurred by health services	Increase in well being in home care group compared to the hospital group shortly after the beginning of care. An annual estimated saving of 34.8% for the home care group compared with the hospital care group
Tsamandouraki (1992) Greece	To compare home care to hospital care	101 hospital patients 101 home care patients	Non-randomised trial	Survival pattern	Significant difference between both groups; better survival in home care care

Table 5.1 Contd.

Author and country	Purpose of the study	Patient population	Study design	Major outcomes	Major results
Ventafridda *et al.* (1989) Italy	To evaluate costs and effectiveness of home care compared to hospital care for advanced cancer patients	60 cancer patients with pain Mean age 59.7	Prospective study of sequential admissions of patients with terminal cancer with pain	Daily recordings of patients on pain intensity and duration, hours of sleep, performance status, side-effects, QoL, costs	Improvement in: performance status and QoL fewer patients feeling very ill less care judged insufficient lower costs No difference in: pain intensity symptoms patients' living conditions relationship with GP
Vincinguerra *et al.* (1986) USA	To compare home care by a multidisciplinary health team with hospital care	44 hospital patients 174 home care patients	Prospective evaluation study	Survival Pain control medications Weight changes Dietary intake	Improved survival for home patients related to performance status Decreased narcotic analgesics for home patients Significant difference in body weight More hospital patients classified as underweight

Reference	Aim	Sample	Design	Measures	Results
Viney et al. (1994) Australia	To compare the quality of life of cancer patients dying in palliative care units and in hospitals	183 patients dying of cancer	Prospective comparison study Content analysis blinded	Content analysis of standardised interview transcripts of psychological states: cognitive anxiety scale, depression scale, hostility scales, sociality scale, positive affect scale	Improvement in: expressed more good feelings less indirectly expressed anger less separation and diffuse anxiety No difference in overall QoL
Voltz et al. (1997) USA	To compare hospice and palliative care units in USA, Germany and Japan	159 patients: 91 USA 34 Germany 34 Japan	Survey	Types of therapies Patient characteristics Informed consent Perception of patients with regard to services	Palliative services in all countries USA – 43% non-cancer patients in comparison to 3% in Germany and Japan USA written informed consent, verbal consent in Germany and Japan Patients satisfied with services in three countries
Wakefield & Ashby (1993) Australia	To determine the levels of satisfaction of relatives with terminal care	100 relatives	Retrospective random sample of relatives of adult patients who died from cancer 12–15 months earlier	Telephone interview on patient's condition, symptoms, treatment effectiveness and satisfaction	Improved access to doctors and satisfaction with hospice care Patients cared for at home more likely to die at home Hospice care rated excellent No difference in access and satisfaction with nurses

Table 5.1 Contd.

Author and country	Purpose of the study	Patient population	Study design	Major outcomes	Major results
Zimmer et al. (1984, 1985) USA	To study the effectiveness and acceptability of a home health care team	158 home-bound patients	Randomised controlled trial	National hospice survey, health services utilisation, diary and billing forms, symptom impact profile (SIP), satisfaction, mortality, place of death	Improvements in: fewer days in out of home services mean utilisation rates fewer hospital and nursing home days average cost per day satisfaction satisfaction of caregivers No difference in: morale functional abilities

5.5   Conclusions

When examining the evidence presented in this chapter on the effectiveness of palliative care models, one is led to believe that palliative care has had some impact on improving outcomes. A number of studies showed improvement in pain and symptom management and in quality of life, in increasing patient and family satisfaction with care, and in reducing costs. There is evidence to suggest that conventional care alone is inadequate in meeting the needs of terminally ill patients and their families. The review also points out that a multiprofessional palliative care team can be very effective in meeting the needs of patients and their families and in providing access to other services at home.

Conducting research in this field is rather complex. A number of limitations and difficulties associated with carrying out research in palliative care need to be taken into consideration when reviewing this evidence. Although randomised controlled trials are the gold standard in assessing effectiveness, they are rare in this field. In addition, difficulties encountered in prospective studies dealing with dying patients are quite common, and as such should not be underestimated. Observational and retrospective studies with carers are as a result more often carried out. The problems and pitfalls of conducting research in this growing field are discussed at greater length in Chapter 10.

Chapter 6

Evaluation of Palliative Care Services: Views of Home Carers and Health Professionals

Huda Huijer Abu-Saad

6.1 Introduction

It is generally accepted that palliative care services should meet the needs of the patients with advanced and incurable disease, their family members and friends, as well as the large number of professional carers. Caring for the carers is an important aspect of palliative care which needs to be addressed and evaluated on a regular basis if quality care is to be provided.

6.2 Views of home carers

People who are terminally ill spend in general as much as 90% of their time at home. Home is usually where people would like to be when ill and where they would like to die. There is a great deal of literature on the effect of caring on people's lives, which includes the financial, emotional and psychological costs encountered as well as the social and employment opportunities forgone (Robbins, 1998). The effects of care giving depict a range of negative responses such as anxiety, exhaustion, stress, strain, health-related problems, financial hardship and role conflicts. The positive responses are nevertheless also commonly cited and include a sense of challenge, providing family cohesiveness, and finding more purpose in life (Herth, 1993).

Studies addressing home carers' satisfaction with care and focusing on needs assessment are of particular importance in palliative care research. In a study focusing on patient-carer dyads using interviews, observations and chart reviews before and after treatment and during rehabilitation, Mah and Johnston (1993) found concerns to vary between patients and their carers across the three time periods. This study points to the need for research that undertakes to delineate the needs of patients and their immediate carers.

Qualitative research methods have been extensively used to address the home carers' needs and concerns. Most of these studies, however, are retrospective and are based on the methodology developed by Cartwright and Seale (1990). Death certificates are in essence used to determine the sample to be included, and family members 6–12 months following bereavement were involved. Interview schedules based on the 'life before death' model are quite popular and have been used by numerous researchers in the UK (Field *et al.* 1992; Addington-Hall & McCarthy, 1995a,b). The strength of this model lies in getting detailed information on the perceptions of the carer of the weeks preceding death, and is relatively free of bias. The weakness of this approach lies in the extent to which carers can give an accurate account of the patients' feelings and experiences with the approaching death.

A study conducted by Addington-Hall *et al.* (1991) on the needs of family carers in the hospital found areas of dissatisfaction to include inadequate symptom control, difficulties in obtaining information, and lack of adequate community services. These results were confirmed by Field *et al.* (1992) who suggested that carers may not be receiving as much contact with the staff as they should, given the goals of the staff to meet the psychosocial needs of patients as well as the carers. In both studies, however, carers remained highly satisfied with the care provided. Kristjanson *et al.* (1996) speculated that family care satisfaction might be the difference between what a person expects and what he or she perceives as being given. Based on this theory, a scale measuring family satisfaction with advanced cancer care was developed and tested in a number of studies (Kristjanson *et al.* 1996). The problems usually encountered with these structured methods of needs assessment and satisfaction with care, concern the extent to which home carers are able to comment on their own feelings and their ability to reflect on the needs and concerns of the patient.

Fakhoury *et al.* (1997), in a study looking at the effects of clinical characteristics of dying patients and the caregivers' satisfaction with palliative care, found more than half (52%) of the informal caregivers to be highly satisfied with the care provided by community nurses. This was in comparison with 39% and 35% of high satisfaction with services provided by general practitioners and hospital doctors respectively. Informal caregivers of patients who died from a lymphatic or haematopoietic tissue cancer were more likely to report satisfaction with hospital doctors. The least satisfaction was reported by caregivers of patients who died from genito-urinary or respiratory and intrathoracic neoplasms. The duration of pain was not related to any of the satisfaction measures. Based on the results the authors recommended that clinical characteristics are taken into consideration in population-based evaluation studies in palliative care. More research into the reasons for dissatisfaction is also warranted.

In a study conducted by Grande *et al.* (1997a,b), the needs for support and the problems in the introduction of support to terminally ill patients and their carers were studied. The study used semi-structured interviews to collect information from patients and their carers as well as a survey to collect data from general practitioners. Results identified special needs mainly in transport, personal care and housework. Reassurance of carers by health professionals was also identified. The balance of needing outside help and keeping one's independence, dignity and familiar aspects of life was also signalled. In addition there may be reluctance from the patients and carers to seek help because of a perceived lack of resources and impingement on health professionals' time. This study points out the importance of introducing services that meet the patients' and carers' needs.

Research issues

Due to the difficulties, methodological and ethical, in conducting research on dying patients, patient surrogates or proxies have been commonly used in palliative care research. It is of particular interest to find out whether patients and home carers tell the same story when reporting the experience with terminal illness, or whether their accounts reflect a different version of the story. These concerns have become issues in palliative care research mainly because some researchers question the ethics of involving dying patients as subjects of research. In the multitude of studies conducted to look at patient/home carer/staff perspective on terminal illness, a high level of congruency was present over symptoms and problems. Home carers tend, however, to report higher levels of patient anxiety and distress than patients themselves, and staff members tend to assess pain to be less severe than patients and home carers. Home carers' accounts in general tend to be less informative and less congruent when assessing the patients' quality of life and when determining the presence of anxiety and depression felt by the patient. For more information on studies of congruency of results, see Robbins (1998).

Not only are the components of palliative care different from standard medical care but so too are the approaches to evaluating palliative care using satisfaction measures. Most satisfaction studies use in general prospective research methods. This is in contrast to evaluation studies in palliative care, the majority of which use retrospective methodologies. Proxies report in general less satisfaction with medical care than the patients themselves (Epstein *et al.*, 1989). Family members in general rate patients' health more negatively than patients do. In addition, in several studies patients and informal carers' perspectives on the quality of palliative care were found to be different (Cartwright & Seale, 1990; Ahmedzai *et al.*, 1991; Hinton, 1996). There is also evidence suggesting that bereaved people's memories and perceptions are affected by depression, with negative memories becoming more accessible than pleasant ones (Bradley *et al.*, 1996). There is also a positive association found between bereaved people's health status and the retrospective evaluation of palliative care services (Fakhoury *et al.*, 1997).

Some people argue as well that expectations about care determine to a large extent patient satisfaction with care. There is empirical evidence suggesting that the higher the number of met expectations the more patients are satisfied with care. This points to the importance of conducting research on identifying and comparing expectations and aspirations of dying patients with those of their carers. Different models of satisfaction with palliative care for patients and carers in palliative care are recommended (Fakhoury, 1998). Multidimensional models of satisfaction that take into account the patients' and carers' views and experiences are much needed if adequate and accurate evaluation of palliative care services is to be achieved.

6.3   Views of professional carers

The evaluation of palliative care services remains incomplete if the views of the health professional carers are not included. The type of work carried out, the competency levels required, how the work is evaluated by parties concerned, and the efficiency of the organisational structure are questions that need to be addressed in palliative care research. The literature provides little information on what the specialist palliative care staff actually do. This is in sharp contrast to the abundance of information on what palliative care staff should do in terms of guidelines, protocols and standards. Very few studies address the actual process of care and the interaction between the professional carers and the terminally ill patients and their families. Observational and descriptive research, in addition to chart reviews, could provide a source of information underpinning evaluative research in this area.

Home care nurses provide to a large extent the greatest volume of palliative care. In addition to domiciliary work, they work either from an inpatient hospice unit or as members of hospital teams. The Macmillan nurses in the UK are usually attached to conventional community nursing teams or to specialist palliative care teams (Boyd, 1992). The role of the nurse includes the provision of advice on symptom control and on psychosocial issues. There is, however, a wide difference in the actual hands-on care provided by the different types of nurses involved in palliative care (Robbins *et al.* 1994). The actual process of care carried out by nurses has been described in two research studies conducted in the UK and Finland (Perakyla, 1989; Hunt, 1991). Both studies identified four main nursing roles in palliative care:

(1)   The bureaucratic/practical role
(2)   The biomedical/medical role
(3)   The social-therapy/psychosocial role
(4)   The friendly, informal/lay role.

Nurses tend to move between the different roles depending on the needs of the patients and their immediate families. Most of the studies conducted on the processes of care are done using nurses as health providers. No studies have been found involving other disciplines as providers of care. As a result more studies involving an interdisciplinary team are warranted.

A postal survey by Hatcliff *et al.* (1996) evaluated the wish of district nurses to provide high quality palliative care at home. A lack of knowledge and experience in, for example, symptom management as well as the size of caseload and time constraints can be regarded as barriers to the provision of high quality palliative care.

Other areas of research warranting more attention are the needs of staff working in palliative care settings. In that respect caring for the professional carers should be given due attention. Vachon *et al.* (1995), in a review of the literature on stress in hospice and palliative care, concluded that high levels of stress among staff were commonly found and have been a matter of concern since the start of the hospice movement. Interventions developed to address stress in palliative care have been successful in lowering the stress levels among palliative care nurses in comparison with nurses working in hospital settings such as intensive care. The same results were found by Graham *et al.* (1996) in a study among UK physicians working in palliative care settings. Support provided to staff working in palliative care services can include different strategies varying from support by friends and colleagues, team-building, continuing education programmes and skill training, to the provision of stress-reduction programmes organised on a regular basis for all staff members. The success of these programmes has been based on descriptive rather than comparative studies. The effectiveness of such stress-reduction programmes has not been adequately evaluated and hence deserves more attention in future studies.

The views of professional carers are without doubt important when palliative care services are under evaluation. Thus the congruence between the patients' reports and professional carers' reports assumes a central place. A number of studies have been conducted addressing this issue. In general, staff rate symptoms as less severe than patients do (Butters *et al.*, 1993; Higginson & McCarthy, 1993) and anxiety and communication problems more severe (Higginson & McCarthy, 1993). Ferrel *et al.* (1993), based on qualitative analysis, showed the differences between staff and patients with regard to pain to be related to different factors. Patients saw pain as a multilayered phenomenon reflecting ultimate and immediate concerns. Patients viewed pain as a challenge with which they had to live and used the severity of pain to monitor the progression of their disease. Nurses, on the other hand, are challenged by the clinical aspects of pain management; pain is perceived as clinically unnecessary for the patient to experience, yet it remains for them a challenge to eradicate.

6.4   Conclusions

In conclusion, there is little evidence in the literature in support of the actual needs of home carers and the actual work of the different types of health professionals in palliative care. There is also very little evidence which points to the impact of what they do on specified patient outcomes. This is not entirely surprising since the process of palliative care is more difficult to observe let alone quantify using observable measures. Nevertheless this area remains of particular importance in evaluating palliative care services. Qualitative research may be the method of choice in this respect, which will help disentangle the meaning of the palliative care experience and of symptom control for the patient, for the home carer and for the health professional. It will be vital in shedding more light on the 'black box' of care provided in this area.

Chapter 7

Pain and Symptom Management

Huda Huijer Abu-Saad and *Annemie Courtens*

7.1 Introduction

This chapter provides an overview of studies on 'total pain' management and symptom management. Attention is first given to the prevalence of symptoms in palliative care. A number of intervention studies addressing symptom management in general and pain management in particular are then addressed. Special attention is given in Chapter 8 to the prevalence of pain and symptom management in children and to intervention studies conducted on this subject.

7.2 Symptom prevalence in palliative care

Since the alleviation of suffering is considered to be one of the main aims of palliative care, adequate treatment of distress due to physical symptoms is a major priority in this field. Symptom distress and requests for treatment are highly prevalent in the last year of life. Prevalence of severe symptoms in advanced cancer patients, including pain, is high ranging between 20% and 60% (Addington-Hall *et al.*, 1992). A number of studies report a prevalence of 60–80% of untreated patients in the last year of life (Levy, 1996; Vainio & Auvinen, 1996; Higginson & Hearn, 1997). In a primary care setting 66% of the patients found the pain in the last year of life to be distressing and 61% experienced distressing pain in the last weeks of life (Addington-Hall & McCarthy, 1995a,b). Based on prevalence studies a total of 16 symptoms experienced by terminal patients have been reported: pain, nausea, vomiting, diarrhoea, confusion, constipation, anorexia, dyspnoea, coughing, sleep disturbances, fatigue, dry mouth, thirst, urinary incontinence, dysphagia and depressed mood. However, when the search is limited to symptoms with 10% or higher prevalence, only 10 symptoms remain: pain, nausea, vomiting, diarrhoea, constipation, anorexia, dyspnoea, cough, sleep disturbances and fatigue (Reuben *et al.*, 1988; Dorrepaal, 1989; Addington-Hall *et al.*, 1991; Cleeland *et al.*, 1994; Addington-Hall & McCarthy 1995a,b; Maltoni *et al.*, 1995; Vainio & Auvinen, 1996; Conill *et al.*, 1997; Lobchuk *et al.*1997).

Asthenia may be considered a common symptom in terminal cancer. It is strongly associated with malnutrition and other tumour-related symptom complexes. Asthenia includes three other major symptoms: fatigue defined as easy tiring and decreased capacity to maintain performance, generalised weakness and mental fatigue (Doyle *et al.*, 1998). Prevalence percentages found for asthenia were over 60% in the reported studies (Bruera *et al.*, 1987; Coyle *et al.*, 1990; Ventafridda *et al.*, 1990; Chan & Woodruff, 1991; Bruera *et al.*, 1993; Donnelly & Walsh, 1995; Conill *et al.*, 1997). Bruera *et al.* (1987) found a prevalence of 72% ($n = 54$) among patients with advanced carcinoma of the breast. Donnelly & Walsh (1995) reported a prevalence of 64% ($n = 1000$) in advanced cancer patients. Another study of Bruera *et al.* (1993) showed 90% ($n = 275$) of the patients with advanced cancer suffering asthenia. Ventafridda *et al.* (1990) showed somewhat different findings of weakness (51%) in terminal cancer patients. Coyle *et al.* (1990) found somewhat similar percentages of generalised weakness ranging from 43 to 49% in terminally ill cancer patients. The percentages of fatigue in the study of Coyle *et al.* (1990) ranged from 52% to 58% at four weeks and one week before death respectively. Conill *et al.* (1997) assessed the symptoms of 176 cancer patients in the last week of their life and compared these prevalences with those of six weeks before. Asthenia was one of the three most frequent symptoms in both periods; prevalence of 77% six weeks before death, and 82% in the last week was found.

Findings on the prevalence of anorexia in advanced cancer vary. Chan and Woodruff (1991) assessed palliative care in a hospital setting and found 42% of terminal cancer patients suffering anorexia. Bruera *et al.* (1993) found a prevalence of 64%, Ng & von Gunten (1998) 44%, Morita *et al.* (1999) 57–95% and Donnelly & Walsh (1995) a prevalence of 85% in advanced cancer patients. The prevalence figures of nausea reported in the reviewed studies differ too. Bruera *et al.* (1993) found nausea in 68% of advanced cancer patients. The findings of a prospective study on symptom prevalence in advanced cancer patients carried out by Donnelly & Walsh (1995) showed nausea in 36% of patients. Findings of the National Hospice Study demonstrated 44% of terminally ill patients with nausea (Reuben & Mor, 1987). Morita *et al.* (1999) identified nausea in 29–48% of terminally ill hospice patients. Ng and von Gunten (1998) found a prevalence rate of 63% in patients admitted to a hospice or palliative care unit. In a study by Ventafridda *et al.* (1990) a very low figure of 6% was found. Coyle *et al.* (1990) also found very low percentages, of approximately 12%, in terminally ill cancer patients.

Depression is a frequent complication of patients with advanced cancer (Lynch, 1995). In the literature review published by Payne (1998) on depression in palliative care, 12 empirical studies were found between 1992 and 1996. A total number of 1163 patients were included in the study. The prevalence of depression in palliative care patients has been found to vary from 3% to 69% (Payne, 1998). The variability in prevalence rates could be related to type of neoplasm, therapy and variations in the diagnostic criteria and measures used. The majority of these studies used cross-sectional designs that provide information on prevalence but not on trends over the dying trajectory. Therefore it is not known to what extent patients become more or less depressed as death approaches (Payne, 1998).

There are indications that female patients report higher levels of distress than male patients, that patients with more advanced disease stages report severe symptom distress, and those with expressed desire for death have a higher frequency of depression (Chochinov *et al.*, 1995; Lynch, 1995).

Constipation is a frequent and distressing complication in terminally ill patients. It is a commonly encountered symptom in the palliative care setting. About 50% of patients admitted to British hospices complain about it. Conill *et al.* 1997 found prevalence percentages of 49% six weeks before death and 55% in the last week of life. In the study of Ng and von Gunten (1998) 50% of the hospice-admitted patients were constipated. Vainio & Auvinen (1996) found a prevalence figure of 23% irrespective of differences among primary sites of cancer. In Bruera and Neumann's (1998) study with 275 cancer patients a prevalence of 65% was found.

Constipation is characterised usually by diminished frequency of defecation associated with difficulty or discomfort. Many patients develop this symptom as a result of opioid therapy but other constipating factors might be intestinal obstruction due to a tumour, hypercalcaemia, inadequate food-intake, weakness, inactivity or confusion (Doyle *et al.*, 1998)

Differences between prevalence figures may be based on differences between methods, populations and time of measurement. Population-based follow-up studies are needed to document the incidence and prevalence of symptoms. Standardised and valid measurement tools and staging systems would improve the comparability of results. Few studies have been carried out on the prevalence of these symptoms in terminally ill patients. Prevalence estimates between the studies differ for most of the examined symptoms. Differences in patient groups, small sample sizes, different measures, and limited data collection periods might cause this. In addition, a number of factors may contribute to the prevalence of symptoms.

Morita *et al.* (1999) performed a prospective study to identify contributing factors to symptoms in terminally ill hospice inpatients and concluded that clinicians can predict the probability of future symptoms based on patients' characteristics, disease state and medication intake. The results of this study showed a number of factors contributing to symptom prevalence in terminally ill cancer patients. These included:

- Young age (pain, abdominal swelling, dry mouth)
- Performance status (anorexia, general malaise, oedema, dyspnoea)
- Brain tumour (paralysis)
- Neoplasms of lung/pleura (dyspnoea, cough/sputum, death rattle)
- Bone metastasis (pain, paralysis)
- Gastric/pancreas cancer (abdominal swelling)
- Peritoneal metastasis (general malaise, oedema, nausea/vomiting, abdominal swelling, dry mouth)
- Opioids (constipation, dry mouth, myoclonus)
- Anticholinergics (dry mouth)
- Antidopaminergics (myoclonus).

The authors suggest that through the identification of factors that could predict the possibility of future suffering, one could probably improve palliative care delivery.

Another issue is the question whether patients or caregivers should be asked about symptoms of patients. Grande *et al.* (1997a) compared the report of symptoms by terminally ill patients with reports by the attending general practitioners. In this survey general practitioners tended to underestimate symptom prevalence when compared with patients. General practitioners reported pain in approximately 66% of the patients, compared with 80% reported by the patients. In a descriptive study by Curtis & Fernsler (1989) pain reports of patients were compared with those of primary caregivers. Patients reported significantly less pain than primary caregivers did. The discrepancy in the reported pain may be related also to the method used; different measures used could lead to different reports of pain.

Impact of symptoms

Severe symptoms in the terminally ill have been shown to impact on functional status and well being (Morris & Sherwood, 1987; Cleeland *et al.*, 1994; Ingham & Protenoy, 1996), to aggravate anxiety and depression (Spiegel *et al.*, 1994; Cleeland *et al.*, 1996), and to affect the patient's wish to die earlier (Toverud Severson, 1997). In a study examining the emotional and social consequences of cancer pain, Strang (1992) found the intensity of pain to be significantly related to an increase in anxiety and depressive feelings and thoughts. Also physical, mental and social activities were affected by pain. Some social activities such as 'spending less time on hobbies' or 'isolating oneself by not going outdoors' significantly correlated with pain intensity. In other words, increased pain led to a decrease in social activities.

Under-treatment of symptoms

Under-treatment of symptoms in the terminal phase has been associated with under-reporting, especially in the case of pain and fatigue (Morris & Sherwood, 1987; Grossman *et al.*, 1991; Cleeland *et al.*, 1994; Ingham & Protenoy, 1996). Several studies (Max, 1990; Wilkie & Keefe, 1991; McCaffery, 1992; Ward *et al.*, 1993) cited a number of patient-related barriers to management of cancer pain. The majority of the patients in their studies denied having pain and other symptoms; they feared the adverse effects of opioids in pain management such as addiction and tolerance. Some patients expressed fatalism whereas others wanted to be seen as a good patient.

Physician-related factors for under-treatment are also comparable to those of patients and are usually related to insufficient symptom assessment and fear of opioids (Von Roenn *et al.*, 1993; Grande *et al.*, 1997a). In addition, competence, knowledge and clinical experience of the physician have been found to play a major role in the treatment modalities used (Grande *et al.*, 1997a). A retrospective study conducted by Chan and Woodruff (1991) on cancer patients in an Australian hospital showed that one third of the patients had inadequate pain relief. This finding was related to lack of medical expertise in using analgesics for chronic cancer pain. Boekema *et al.* (1994) studied the effectiveness of pain control among general practitioners and medical specialists in the Netherlands. Results showed a moderate satisfaction of both disciplines with pain measures used, with the diagnostic possibilities available and with the effectiveness of treatments employed in pain control. Boekema *et al.* (1994) concluded, based on the results of their study, that emphasis needed to be placed on co-ordination, co-operation and communication in transmural cancer care.

Symptom management

Symptom monitoring by patients is often used to enhance symptom management and improve care. The monitoring of symptoms is often carried out using four axes: severity, distress, treatment requests and treatment effect. The effectiveness of symptom monitoring is enhanced if it is detailed, clinically relevant and directly applicable to clinical practice. Symptom severity is of primary importance in symptom management and as such should be simple, straightforward, valid and responsive to change in palliative care. Symptom management can be improved by providing the physicians with the necessary knowledge and skills through continuing education programmes and courses in skill assessment and monitoring. Other methods include strengthening the role of the patient, providing support from specialised home care nurses, using patient diaries for continuous monitoring and using appropriate patient educational materials such as information booklets, flyers, audiotapes etc. (Rinck *et al.*, 1997; de Wit & van Dam, 1997). The symptom assessment/monitoring tools completed by the patients can be used to provide feedback on a regular basis to the health professionals. They can then be incorporated in the clinical decision-making during each professional caregiver–patient encounter.

For pain, dyspnoea, nausea and vomiting, anorexia, fatigue, delirium, constipation and depression, some issues on assessment and management will be described in the next section.

7.3   Assessment and management of pain

Bonica (1985), a pioneer in the field of cancer pain, has provided some of the early reports on cancer pain prevalence. Depending on the type of neoplasm, Bonica found pain to be experienced by 20–50% of patients when the lesion was diagnosed, by nearly half of the patients in the prevalence group, and by 55–95% of the patients with far advanced or terminal cancer. The results pointed out in addition that pain was experienced as moderate to severe in 50% of the patients and very severe or excruciating in 30% of the studied population. Coyle *et al.* (1990), in a study conducted at the Memorial Sloan-Ketering Cancer Centre in the USA, found that 100% of the patients included in the survey had pain. In

67% of the patients, a combination of more than one type of pain was present; somatic and neuropathic pain occurred in 40% of the patients. In the four-week interval before death, pain was described by 80% of the patients to be moderate and by 20% as severe. Pooled data reported recently suggest that cancer pain is reported by about 50% of patients at all stages of the disease and by over 70% of patients with advanced neoplasms (see Table 7.1). In addition, the data emphasise that pain prevalence in the community is as high as that observed in other settings and that multidisciplinary palliative care teams are effective in alleviating pain (Higginson & Hearn, 1997).

In a compelling editorial on chronic pain, Gallagher (1998) asserts that pain is not only an aggressive disease that damages the nervous system but also an aggressive social disease that attacks one's psychological state and social coping. The anguish of suffering with pain in the context of not being believed and socially supported is speculated to chronically activate the neurophysiological systems associated with pain intensity. In other words it may facilitate pain transmission, sensitise nociceptors and activate neuropathic pain.

Kuuppelomaki & Lauri (1998) using qualitative research methodologies described the nature and content of the experiences of suffering of patients with incurable cancer. Three different dimensions were identified in patients' experiences of suffering; physical, psychological and social. The primary sources of physical suffering were found to be fatigue, pain and the side effects of chemotherapy. The causes of psychological suffering were found to be related to the physiological changes associated with the disease and the imminence of death and were mostly manifested in depression. Social suffering was related to the deterioration of the disease and the fear of infections, restricting patients from maintaining social contacts.

Pain assessment

An expert working group of the European Association of Palliative Care (Caraceni *et al.*, 2000) has been active in developing guidelines to standardise pain measurement and assessment tools in palliative care. This section will be based on the working party's recommendations in this area.

Pain is defined by many as a subjective sensation that can be described using relevant features or attributes (quality, location, intensity, duration, frequency, aversiveness, emotional reaction and physical and psychosocial impact). Among these attributes, intensity is recognised as one of the most relevant clinical dimensions of the pain experience. Being a subjective experience there is no objective method or gold standard by which to measure pain. A number of unidimensional self-report tools, however, have been developed and tested to measure pain in a reliable and valid way.

Three types of unidimensional pain measurement tools were found to be valid and reliable and appropriate for use in palliative care (Caraceni *et al.*, 2000). These include visual analogue scales (VAS), categorical verbal rating scales (VRS) and categorical numerical rating scales (NRS).

Table 7.1 Pain prevalence.

Authors	Type of study	Number	Country	Percentage with pain	Stage cancer	Setting
Trotter et al. (1981)	Prospective study	237	UK	72	Advanced	Outpatient clinic
Spiegel & Bloom (1983)	Prospective study	86	USA	56	Advanced	Outpatient clinic
Bonica (1985)		2750	USA	68	Advanced/terminal	Review of 13 reports
Mor (1987)	Prospective study	2046	USA	68	Terminal	Hospices
Ventafridda et al. (1990)	Cross-sectional study	115	Italy	59	Terminal	Outpatient clinic; hospital; at home
Coyle et al. (1990)	Survey	90	USA	100	Terminal	At home referred to a supportive care team
Addington-Hall et al. (1992)	Randomised control trial	203	UK	53–56	Terminal	Inner London health district
Donnelly & Walsh (1995)	Prospective studies	1000	USA	82	Advanced	Inpatients and outpatients
Ellershaw (1995)	Prospective study	125	UK	74	Advanced	Hospital team
Vainio & Auvinen (1996)	Prospective study	1640	USA, UK, Finland, Australia, Switzerland	51	Advanced/terminal	40 palliative care centres
Grande et al. (1997a)	Survey	30	UK	80	Terminal	Family Health Services Authority register in Cambridgeshire
Higginson & Hearn (1997)	Prospective study	695 Irish, 277 English	England and Ireland	70	Advanced	Specialist home care services and hospice referrals

Visual analogue scale (VAS)

The VAS is an unmarked line with extreme descriptors of no pain and worst pain. Patients are usually asked to mark the segment of the line that best describes their pain experience:

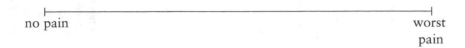

no pain   worst
                                                                                                                      pain

Verbal rating scale (VRS)

A VRS represents a sequence of words describing different intensity levels of pain. A commonly used version of a verbal rating scale is:

None   mild   moderate   severe

Numeric rating scale (NRS)

The NRS can be seen as a variation of the VAS using numbers or gradations that indicate the severity of the subjective pain experience:

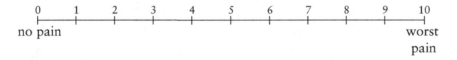

no pain   worst
                                                                                                                      pain

Evidence suggests that numeric rating scales are easier to apply and are associated with better compliance than VAS and VRS. Although all three scales are typically administered in a pencil and paper format, other valid approaches for VAS and NRS include the use of touch screens, sliding scales and verbal administration.

In addition to the above scales measuring the intensity of pain, empirical evidence on self-monitoring of pain using a pain diary has been tested in terminally ill cancer patients at home (de Wit *et al.*, 1999a). The results showed the pain diary to be appropriate for use in assessing cancer patients' pain intensity at home. Despite the fact that many patients were in bad health, patients' compliance with the pain diary was very high. Patients reported that through the pain diary they gained better insight into their pain experience, giving them in some respect a sense of control over their pain and ways to deal with it.

Because pain is a multidimensional construct, the assessment of the multitude of factors impinging on the pain experience becomes imperative. The expert working group recommends the use of two multidimensional scales in palliative care: the short form of the Brief Pain Inventory (BPI) and the McGill Pain Questionnaire (MPQ). Both of these tools are well validated in multiple languages and are thus suitable for application in an international setting (Caraceni *et al.*, 2000).

The Brief Pain Inventory is a simple and easily administered tool that provides information on pain history, intensity, location and quality. Numeric scales (range 0 to 10) indicate the intensity of pain in general, at its worst, at its least and right now. A percentage scale quantifies relief from current therapies. A figure representing the body is provided for the patient to shade the area corresponding to his or her pain. Seven questions determine the degree to which pain interferes with function, mood and enjoyment of life. The BPI is self administered and easily understood, and has been translated into many languages.

The McGill Pain Questionnaire (MPQ) is a self-administered questionnaire that provides global scores and subscale scores that reflect the sensory, affective and evaluative dimensions of pain. The scale has been validated in cancer pain. A short form of the MPQ (SF-MPQ) consists of 15 representative words from the sensory ($n = 11$) and affective ($n = 4$) categories of MPQ. The BPI verbal rating scale and a visual analogue scale (VAS) measuring pain intensity are included. The 15 words are scored using a four-point verbal rating scale, ranging from none, mild and moderate to severe pain. The SF-MPQ correlates highly with the MPQ. While the MPQ is available in many languages the SF-MPQ is not.

In studying the effectiveness of pain relief, patients are asked, using the intensity scales for instance, to compare pain now with pain prior to commencing pain therapies. Adequacy of pain treatment can be based in general on either patient-oriented measures such as pain intensity markers, pain relief scales and patient satisfaction scales, or a pain score related to the pain medication as provided by clinicians, such as pain management indexes (de Wit *et al.*, 1999b; de Wit *et al.*, 2000a). To identify changes in cancer pain treatments and to describe the effects of specific pain therapies, the development and testing of appropriate pain outcome measures of pain treatments in palliative care remain crucial.

Pain management

In 1982, a WHO consultation in Milan, Italy, brought together a large number of experts in the field of cancer pain. The aim of the meeting was the development of clinical guidelines on the relief of cancer pain. Studies on the applicability of these guidelines have since been carried out under the auspices of WHO in many countries in the world. Since the first meeting in 1982, a number of important consensus meetings have taken place and have resulted in the publication of important documents on cancer pain relief and the WHO three-step analgesic ladder (WHO 1990) (see Fig. 7.1).

A number of studies on controlling pain and symptom management have been reported in the field of palliative care. Ellershaw (1995) studied prospectively 125 patients suffering malignancies and receiving palliative care. In this study 245 pharmacological interventions in symptom control were undertaken, 160 relating to pain control and 85 to control of other symptoms. A palliative care assessment tool (PACA) was used to assess the outcome of interventions. The PACA tool comprised a four-point scale to describe the severity of the symptoms from the patient's perspective, using a semi-structured interview. In controlling pain the major intervention was initiation and adjustment of opioid, anti-inflammatory and anti-neuralgic analgesic medication. Results showed

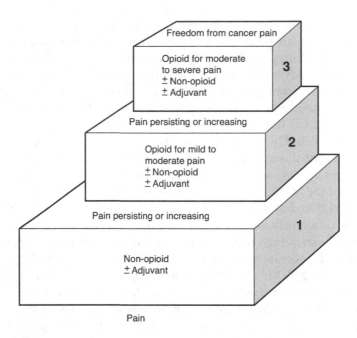

Fig. 7.1 WHO analgesic ladder (WHO, 1998).

significant improvements in the control of pain. The number of patients in whom pain dominated daily life reduced from 30% to 7%.

Ventafridda *et al.* (1990) conducted a cross-sectional study using 115 terminal cancer patients who had been undergoing palliative care during a single week at the outpatient clinic, in hospital or at home. Assessment took place with a weekly descriptive self-report. The number of patients treated with strong opioids increased from 25% to 74% during palliative treatment. Similar to Ellershaw (1995), Ventafridda *et al.* (1990) found less pain in terminally ill patients after initiating palliative care treatment. The percentage of patients with pain diminished significantly from 59% to 35%. A prospective study of Higginson & Hearn (1997) carried out in community- and hospital-based palliative care settings in the UK and Ireland examined pain control in 695 terminal cancer patients. Pain was recorded using body charts. One item of the support team assessment schedule was used at referral and then weekly to rate the severity of the pain. Two weeks after referral to palliative care services, pain control had led to a significant reduction in the levels of pain experienced by the patients. Pain was reduced from 33% to 20% in the patients suffering moderate pain and from 11% to 4% among patients with severe pain.

A nationwide survey by Hiraga *et al.* (1991) in Japan showed the rate of pain relief in the terminal stage to be improved. The propagation of WHO-advocated cancer pain therapeutics might be responsible for this. The rate of complete pain relief proved to be significantly higher among patients hospitalised in adult disease/cancer centres than for those hospitalised in university hospitals. The rate of pain relief rose from 37.8% in 1986 to 43.9% in 1990 with a peak in 1988 of

48.6%. In order to relieve pain, non-steroid anti-inflammatory agents (NSAIDS) including paracetamol and aspirin, agonist-antagonists such as pentazocine and buprenorphine, and morphine or parenterally injected opioids were used. Chan and Woodruff (1991) studied the medical records of 110 hospitalised patients with terminal cancer. Pain was improved in 66% ($n = 110$) of the patients, 33% receiving inadequate pain relief. Analgesics used were strong opioid analgesics (morphine, methadone), weak opioid analgesics such as codeine, oxycodone and dextropropoxyphene, and also non-opioid analgesics like aspirin, paracetamol and non-steroidal anti-inflammatory drugs. Furthermore, pain treatment included non-pharmacological forms such as radiotherapy, intercostal nerve blocks and rhizotomy.

Baumann *et al.* (1986) evaluated in a pilot study the effects of patient-controlled analgesia (PCA) in terminally ill cancer patients. Eight patients whose pain was not adequately controlled by oral narcotics used PCA for 48 hours. Respiratory rates, sedation and pain outcome measures indicated that these patients achieved satisfactory analgesia with minimum sedation and experienced no respiratory depression. PCA, using a self-dosing technique, was judged to be safe, effective and able to accommodate a wide range of fluctuations in analgesic use in terminally ill patients in pain. In a study by Boersma *et al.* (1989), terminally ill cancer patients with very severe or unbearable pain were treated with epidural sufentanil. The patients remained in the hospital for two to three days to titrate the infusion rate and to monitor the effectiveness of pain relief and any possible side effects before discharge home. In the home situation, patients were supervised by their general practitioner. The majority of the patients had epidural sufentanil until they died. Pain relief was effective with no reported infections or respiratory depression. The authors concluded that epidural sufentanil infusion was a safe and effective method for pain control in terminally ill patients at home.

In a review article on the use of opioids in advanced malignant disease, Boisvert and Cohen (1995) concluded that there is a wide variation in mean daily dose of opioids used. They warn clinicians of the adverse effects of high doses, as they are associated with higher toxicity and more costs. The authors recommend that reporting of cancer pain and pharmacological and non-pharmacological interventions for patients be standardised in order to allow for rational guidelines to be established for opioid use in advanced cancer.

The use of non-pharmacological pain-relief techniques has been advocated in palliative care. Most cognitive-behavioural interventions have been studied in chronic non-cancer pain patients. Interventions in cancer patients primarily concentrated on increasing patients' knowledge and increasing compliance with medication prescriptions. Patient education and empowerment of patients to take an active role in their pain treatments form the cornerstones of effective pain management. In spite of the importance of patient education in pain control, very few studies have been conducted in this area. De Wit *et al.* (2000b), using an experimental longitudinal design, tested the effectiveness of a tailored cognitive-behavioural pain education programme developed for terminally ill cancer patients. The pain education programme was provided in a one-to-one setting lasting between 30 and 60 minutes in the hospital followed by two phone calls at home. Nurses specially trained in cancer pain management gave the education programme. The intervention proved to be feasible. It resulted in a definite increase in patients' pain knowledge and a decrease in experienced pain. The adequacy of pain treatment was also improved as well as the degree of adherence with pain medication. Improved satisfaction with the pain treatment was also found.

An analysis of the music therapy literature yields numerous reports on the effectiveness of music in relieving pain in palliative care. In a graphical analysis of 17 terminally ill patients, Curtis (1986) found perceived pain relief, physical comfort, relaxation and contentment scores to be improved after listening to music. The theoretical underpinnings of these results are related to the psychological relationship between music and pain. Cortical processes are known to influence the intensity and quality of the pain experience through psychological variables such as previous memory of pain, one's understanding of the meaning and origin of pain, cultural factors, one's level of anxiety and distractions as well as personality variables. In this respect music plays a role in providing distraction and reducing anxiety.

Secondly, cognitive coping strategies and the concept that competing stimuli reduce pain perception provide another theoretical perspective. Imagery has been found to be effective, including, 'imagining oneself sitting in comfort and listening to music'. The possibility of listening to music to promote imagery and its effects on pain warrant further investigation.

Thirdly, spinal mechanisms are involved in the modulation of pain. It is possible that music could stimulate brain stem centres either directly via the auditory pathway or by indirect cortical mechanisms that include the psychological/cognitive processes.

Finally, there is the possibility that listening to one's favourite music may cause endorphins to be released in the bloodstream. Goldstein (1980) found that people who experienced 'thrills' in response to their favourite music, experienced fewer thrills when listening to their favourite music after being given a dose of opiate antagonist, naloxone.

7.4   Assessment and management of dyspnoea

Dyspnoea is one of the most frightening and distressing symptoms in the terminal phase. It can be seen as a common cause of suffering for patients in the last months of life. It can result from metastatic malignancy to the lungs or plura, from heart failure, from chest wall weakness due to neuromuscular disease, or from primary pulmonary disease.

McCord and Cronin-Stubbs (1992) as well as Gift (1990) recognised dyspnoea as a multidimensional concept. McCord and Cronin made a distinction of four components:

- Physiological and psychological events or stimuli preceding the development of dyspnoea

- Characteristics of individuals or the environment affecting the response
- Reactions to dyspnoea
- Outcomes that result once the individual has reacted to a stimulus.

To determine the epidemiology of dyspnoea in palliative care Reuben and Mor (1987) used data from the national hospice study, which followed patients during their last six weeks of life. The incidence of dyspnoea was found to be 70% with prevalence rates generally exceeding 50%. According to Ahmedzai (1993a) the incidence of dyspnoea in advanced cancer varies greatly from 29% to 74%. Ripamonti and Bruera (1997) report dyspnoea to occur in 21–78% of cancer patients, days or weeks before death, and to be found difficult to control. Both Heyse-Moore (1991) and Twycross (1993) found that the incidence of dyspnoea increased as death approached and all the studies noted that dyspnoea was the most common severe main symptom in the last days of life. Roberts *et al.* (1993) examined the phenomenon of dyspnoea in the last weeks of life using the experiences of patients themselves and their professional nurse carers. Using a range of descriptive and interpretative approaches, the authors sought to understand how patients and nurses interpret the nature and meaning of this symptom. Results showed that although dyspnoea seemed to be a significant clinical problem for patients in the terminal phase of cancer and in spite of the availability of effective interventions, dyspnoea was often under-reported by patients and unnoticed by health professionals.

What does seem to be well investigated is that the relationship between the magnitude of dyspnoea as perceived by the patient and pulmonary function as an objective measure is inconsistent (van der Molen, 1995). Researchers have found great variability in the expression of dyspnoea among patients with similar functional abnormalities (Bruera & Neumann, 1998). Therefore the goal of treatment in palliative care should be to improve the subjective sensation of the patient rather than trying to modify any abnormalities in blood gases or pulmonary function.

Advances in the management of dyspnoea require assessment tools sensitive enough to effectively measure the outcomes of interventions. Dyspnoea is difficult to quantify because it is a complex, multidimensional and subjective sensation. Dyspnoea does not occur in isolation. Fatigue, depression, anxiety and poor appetite seem to be co-existing factors (van der Molen, 1995) which should be taken into account in instruments that are developed to quantify dyspnoea. Van der Molen (1995) reviewed and analysed the available literature on measurement instruments for assessing breathlessness and their application to patients with advanced cancer.

Several authors used visual analogue scales (Gift, 1989) to measure the perception of the severity of the sensation. Another well-known scale is the modified Borgscale (Burdon *et al.*, 1992) which is an 11-point self-report scale. It is generally used to grade the perception of dyspnoea against exercise testing. According to van der Molen (1995) further work is required to determine what place it has in assessing dyspnoea in advanced cancer. The chronic respiratory disease questionnaire of Guyatt *et al.* (1987) is an instrument that focuses on breathlessness from the patient's point of view and its impact on quality of life. It is developed for patients with chronic pulmonary disease but is demonstrating potential value as an assessment tool for patients with advanced cancer.

Van der Molen (1995) concluded that many of the reviewed instruments have a valuable contribution to make in the assessment of dyspnoea. However, many of the instruments fail to be sensitive enough to detect possible significant changes, are not specific for patients with advanced disease and do not cover all the different components of dyspnoea, i.e. perception, effort and outcome. As a result, more work is needed on the development of specific instruments in this area.

The palliation of cancer-related breathlessness is challenging and complex. A number of methods have been advocated to deal with breathlessness in the terminal phase of illness; few of these methods, however, have been adequately tested.

Bruera *et al.* (1993) in a prospective, double blind, crossover trial studied the effects of supplemental oxygen on the intensity of dyspnoea. Patients were randomised to receive either oxygen or air. The severity of dyspnoea was assessed using a visual analogue scale. Results showed oxygen to be more beneficial than air and moreover it was preferred by patients. Boyd and Kelly (1997) studied in an uncontrolled trial the effects of oral morphine on dyspnoea among patients with advanced cancer. They concluded that regular titrated oral morphine may improve dyspnoea in some patients with advanced cancer but can cause significant short-term effects. Oral morphine can be given to these patients as a therapeutic trial but should be carefully monitored for side effects. Several randomised controlled trials have found that systemic opioid therapy is beneficial for patients with cancer dysnpoea (Bruera & Neumann, 1998). However the optimal type, dose and mode of administration have not yet been determined.

Corner *et al.* (1996) in a randomised controlled trial examined the effectiveness of non-pharmacological interventions for breathlessness in lung cancer. The intervention included weekly sessions by a nurse practitioner using counselling, breathing retraining, relaxation, and teaching coping and adaptation strategies. Results showed significant improvements on breathlessness ratings, distress levels, functional capacity and activities of daily living. No improvements were found for anxiety and depression. Filshie *et al.* (1996), in an open pilot study, explored the efficacy of acupuncture in 20 patients who were breathless at rest. Outcome measures included pulse and respiratory rate, oxygen saturation and patient subjective rating on a visual analogue 'scale of breathlessness, pain, anxiety and relaxation. The majority of the patients reported significant symptomatic benefit from treatment, especially related to breathlessness, anxiety, pain and relaxation as well as significant reductions in heart rate. Based on the results of this pilot study, further research looking at the therapeutic value of acupuncture in the management of breathlessness is warranted.

Several lines of research have provided some evidence that dyspnoea in the terminal phase of life can be adequately managed. Promising areas of research include the use of opioids, respiratory stimulants and oxygen therapy, providing support for respiratory muscles, and nurse-initiated non-pharmacological interventions. Opioids already play a role in managing cancer pain. They moderate the reflexive drive to breathe and thereby decrease patient awareness of dyspnoea. They may also improve breathing efficiency and exercise endurance (Doyle *et al.*, 1993). Support of respiratory muscles is an area deserving further investigation in the management of dyspnoea. Patients with advanced chronic illness often have the cachexia-anorexia syndrome and have lost a great deal of somatic protein. Their diaphragm and the external accessory respiratory muscles may be vulnerable to wasting and fatigue. Improvement in patient nutrition with improvement in respiratory muscle might consequently improve dyspnoea. Finally, an area of particular importance is the effectiveness of non-pharmacological interventions and biofeedback in dyspnoea relief. These areas warrant future investigation in palliative care.

7.5 Assessment and management of fatigue

The first challenge in assessing and managing fatigue is to agree on a definition. The lack of definitional clarity has been attributed by scientists to many factors, among which is the multi-causal and multi-dimensional nature of this phenomenon. Investigators have had difficulties differentiating between fatigue's causes, e.g. anaemia, depression or lack of support; its signs and symptoms, e.g. reduction in force, reduction of activity or concentration or tiredness in whole body; its outcomes, e.g. decreased activity, functional status, capacity, stamina, or endurance; and other signs and symptoms related to fatigue, e.g. weakness, asthenia, malaise and exertion. While it is commonly agreed that fatigue should be viewed as a multidimensional phenomenon, similar to pain in its complexity, fatigue's dimensions have not yet been thoroughly researched or conceptualised.

Most of the studies on fatigue were done using patients undergoing treatment, for instance chemotherapy or radiotherapy (Winningham *et al.*, 1994; Richardson & Ream, 1996). Studies indicate that during the course of chemotherapy 70–100% of the patients experience significant fatigue. Similar prevalence rates (68–100%) have been found in other studies (Smets *et al.*, 1993). Follow-up studies show in addition that most patients remain fatigued long after treatment has ended. In the terminally ill Bruera & Neumann (1998) found a prevalence percentage of 90% and Conill *et al.* (1997) reported 82% in the last week of the patient's life.

Stone *et al.* (1999) reported a study that aimed to determine the prevalence of fatigue among palliative care inpatients compared with a control group without cancer. The prevalence of severe subjective fatigue (defined as fatigue greater than that experienced by 95%'of the control group) in the palliative care population was found to be 75%. The severity of fatigue was unrelated to age, sex, diagnosis, presence or site of metastases, anaemia, dose of opioid or steroid, nutritional status, voluntary muscle function or mood. Kaasa *et al.* (1999) concluded that the level of fatigue was much higher in two palliative care populations as compared to normal population samples and a group of Hodgkin's disease survivors, and that fatigue was almost unchanged over time in the palliative care population.

Significant correlates of fatigue were found to be loss of appetite (Molassiotis *et al.*, 1996), weight loss (Irvine *et al.*, 1994), depression, anxiety, mood disturbance and confusion (Smets, 1997). Stone *et al.* (1999) concluded that fatigue severity was associated with pain and dyspnoea scores. The causes of fatigue remain obscure and further research is required to determine the associations between fatigue and other symptoms.

There are several fatigue scales but there is no universally accepted assessment instrument available. Few of these measures were tested on terminally ill patients.

A common approach to the assessment of fatigue is to use single item self-report measures of either the presence or intensity of fatigue. The Rhoten fatigue scale (Rhoten, 1982), for example, includes a single item ten-point Likert scale on which patients can rate their current level of fatigue. Another is the profile of mood states–fatigue scale (McNair *et al.*, 1981) which measures both presence and intensity of fatigue. These measures do not assess several other important dimensions of fatigue. A simple unitary measure of global fatigue is the nine-item fatigue severity scale (Krupp *et al.*, 1989) which has been tested for validity and reliability by Stone *et al.* (1999) in a palliative setting. There are a few measures designed to consider the multidimensional nature of fatigue: the Piper fatigue scale (Piper *et al.*, 1989), the multidimensional fatigue inventory (Smets *et al.*, 1995) and the fatigue symptom inventory (Hann *et al.*, 1998). The Piper fatigue scale has been found to possess adequate statistical reliability when used in cancer patients. However, no evidence has been presented to support the validity of the scale. In addition, some practical problems have been identified, resulting in the scale hardly being used (Smets, 1997; Hann *et al.*, 1998)

The multidimensional fatigue inventory (MFI) (Smets, 1997) contains 20 items that are divided into five subscales assessing general fatigue, physical fatigue, mental fatigue, reduction in motivation and reduction in activity. The MFI shows good internal consistency and convergent and construct validity. Other psychometric properties require further examination.

Kaasa *et al.* (1999) used the fatigue questionnaire in a palliative population. The fatigue questionnaire was originally developed to measure fatigue among patients with so-called fatigue syndrome and is well validated internationally. It consists of two domains, physical fatigue and mental fatigue, and has 11 items. Kaasa suggests that the content validity of this measure should be further explored in palliative settings.

Fatigue and other symptoms may impose limitations on assessment. The lengths of multidimensional assessment scales may be problematic in this vulnerable patient group. Ongoing research will hopefully focus on the validity, reliability and feasibility of instruments for fatigue in the terminally ill.

Very few studies have tested specific interventions to reduce fatigue among patients. Winningham *et al.* (1994) and Piper (1993) found that fatigue had been reduced through the interventions tested. These results, although isolated, do suggest some avenues to pursue in future research, for example testing the effectiveness of preparatory sensory information, structured support groups, aerobic exercises, drug therapies and attention-restoring activities. None of these interventions have been tested in the terminally ill.

Bruera & Neumann (1998) suggest that in patients with asthenia some general non-pharmacological measures such as adapting the activities of daily living, physiotherapy and occupational therapy, or general pharmacologic measures including corticosteroids and amphetamines, could be used. Corticosteroids have been found to decrease the symptoms of asthenia, either by inhibiting tumour-induced by-products or by inducing a central euphoriant effect. Amphetamines have been found to antagonise opioid induced sedation and fatigue.

7.6 Assessment and management of nausea and vomiting

Nausea and vomiting are among the most distressing adverse effects of cancer chemotherapy (Del Favero *et al.*, 1993) and they are almost universal symptoms of advanced cancer.

Terminal cancer patients report nausea and vomiting with an overall prevalence of 60% and 30% respectively (Mystakidou *et al.*, 1998). Patients with terminal cancer frequently experience nausea for extended periods, often more than four weeks (Bruera & Neumann, 1998). Chemotherapy or radiotherapy, metabolic disturbances, mechanical deformation of the gastrointestinal tract, opioid analgesics or brain metastases are the primary causes in terminal cancer patients. The great majority of research has taken place in the area of che-motherapy-induced emesis. The main reasons for this trend include the dramatic morbidity commonly seen with anti-emetic drugs and the possibility of designing and conducting clinical trials in this area. The last ten years have witnessed considerable advances in the prevention of chemotherapy-induced emesis. The selective 5-hydroxytryptamine (serotonin) inhibitors have been widely and successfully used in the control of emesis (Hainsworth, 1993). Few studies have been conducted, however, in terminally ill cancer patients.

Bruera *et al.* (1994a), in a double blind crossover study that tested the effectiveness of metoclopramide in patients with chronic nausea associated with advanced cancer, concluded that the drug is safe and effective. Bruera concluded from several studies (Bruera *et al.*, 1994a; Bruera, 1996) that slow-release metoclopramide is more effective than the rapid-release formulation and that dexamethasone and other corticosteroids can potentiate the anti-emetic effects of metoclopramide. Mystakidou *et al.* (1998) performed a randomised trial to evaluate the efficacy of tropisetron and chlorpromazine in the management of nausea and vomiting in terminal cancer patients. They concluded that tropisetron is well tolerated and may be the best choice for controlling persistent nausea and vomiting.

Since nausea and vomiting are common and often overlooked causes of impairment in cancer patients, Lindley *et al.* (1992) undertook a study that examined the broad range of consequences associated with emesis related to chemotherapy. Their findings showed a significant decrease in quality of life in patients experiencing nausea and vomiting. These patients reported that vomiting and to a lesser extent nausea substantially influenced their ability to complete household tasks, enjoy meals, spend time with family and friends and maintain daily function and recreation, and thus contributed to a significant change in their quality of life.

Ellershaw (1995) found significant improvements in controlling nausea and anorexia in patients receiving palliative care. Contrary to these results, Ventafridda *et al.* (1990) found nausea to increase from 6% to 9% during palliative treatment. This might be due to palliative treatment with strong opioids in 74% of the patients. Furthermore, a significant decline in feelings of weakness and in depressive feelings was found.

A number of unresolved problems remain, however: identification of the best anti-emetic treatment, optimisation of treatment for the most widely used chemotherapy regimens, and identification of rescue treatment for patients who fail to respond to anti-emetic prophylaxis.

Although chronic nausea is highly prevalent and distressing to terminally ill patients, the understanding of the mechanisms and treatment of this complex and multicausal condition is limited. More studies on the cost effectiveness of emesis relief are still badly needed in the current times of financial constraints. In addition, future research needs to address the impact of both chemotherapy-induced and chronic emesis within the context of other devastating symptom complexes in advanced cancer. The presence of cachexia, chronic pain and cognitive failure may have major influences on the assessment and management of nausea and vomiting in palliative care and therefore warrants attention. There is also a need for an assessment tool for nausea and vomiting. Tools for self-completion by the patient and biological markers of emesis need to be developed and evaluated.

Studies in patients with chemotherapy have shown that patients can learn techniques such as progressive muscle relaxation or guided mental imagery and that they are effective during the stress of chemotherapy. Those techniques might be adapted for nauseated people with advanced disease.

Also transcutaneous electrical nerve stimulation (TENS), acupuncture and acupressure are possible non-drug measures that warrant further exploration (Mannix, in Doyle *et al.*, 1998)

7.7   Assessment and management of anorexia

Anorexia is a highly prevalent symptom among patients with advanced disease. In approximately 80% of the patients this decrease in appetite accompanied by a decrease in food intake is present. Anorexia is a multicausal syndrome being both partially the cause and also partially the consequence of the metabolic changes and the malnutrition that occurs in advanced cancer (Bruera & Fainsinger, in Doyle *et al.*, 1998). Tumour factors, macrophage factors, endogenous peptides and satiens are known to have anorectic effects (Bruera & Fainsinger, in Doyle *et al.*, 1998). Simons (1997) has also mentioned alterations in taste, delayed gastric emptying leading to early satiety and abdominal fullness and learned food aversions as possible causes. Psychological stimuli that might interfere with appetite include anxiety and depression symptoms common in terminally ill patients (Grant & Rivera, 1995). Cognitive failure, also highly prevalent in advanced cancer, may result in patients being unable to prepare or eat their meals. Finally, other symptoms like severe pain, mouth problems, gastrointestinal problems and chronic nausea can make food intake difficult for patients.

Assessment of anorexia may include subjective and objective aspects. The patient's appetite can be quantified by means of a visual analogue scale. Information about anorexia may also be gathered from the patient's family or significant others based on their observations (Grant & Rivera, 1995). Objective evaluation is the analysis of food intake by means of a 1–3 day food intake diary that includes times and amounts of food eaten, calculation of body mass index and other anthropometric evaluations like triceps skinfolds, midarm muscle circumference or laboratory indicators. Interventions for anorexia might be pharmacological or nutritional. Some medications have been used and tested for the treatment of anorexia: megastrol acetate, pentoxifylinne, metoclopramide, cannabinoids, dexamethasone and prednisolone.

Progestational drugs like megestrol acetate and medroxyprogesterone acetate were shown to improve appetite in several randomised trials in terminally ill patients (Bruera *et al*, 1990; Loprinzi *et al.*, 1990; Tchekmedyian *et al*, 1990; Bruera, 1996; Rowland *et al.*, 1996; Simons *et al*, 1996; Beller *et al.* 1997). Side effects that may occur in mostly a mild form are oedema, hypercalcemia and Cushing's syndrome. The high cost of these drugs is a concern, however.

Pentoxifylinne is able to decrease the tumour necrosis factor levels and decrease replication of the AIDS virus. These findings suggest a beneficial role for this drug on cachexia and anorexia. However, double blind, placebo-controlled studies were not able to show any beneficial effect on appetite in cancer patients (Goldberg *et al.*, 1995) or AIDS patients (Dezube *et al.*, 1993). The prokinetic agent metoclopramide has a positive effect on gastric emptying and may have a place in the treatment of anorexia or cachexia. No placebo-controlled studies were found that confirm this possibility. The same conclusion can be made for cannabinoids that increase appetite at the level of the central nervous system but have important disadvantages such as euphoria, dizziness, thinking abnormalities and somnolence (Simons, 1997). In several randomised placebo-controlled trials it was shown that corticosteroids induce an increase – usually temporary – in appetite and improve quality of life (Simons, 1997; Bruera & Neumann, 1998). However, in none of these studies was an effect on weight gain found. The most effective dose and route of administration have not been established and should be addressed in randomised controlled trials. Simons (1997) and Bruera & Neumann (1998) suggest that these drugs can be used among patients who are not expected to live for long and in whom weight gain is not a likely outcome.

A preliminary report of Bruera *et al.* (1999) about the effectiveness of thalidomide among patients with cachexia due to terminal cancer suggests that this drug seems to improve appetite and overall well being. Their preliminary findings suggest also that thalidomide can be expected to be well tolerated and to have at least similar symptomatic effects as megastrol acetate. Further research needs to be conducted to better understand the possible effects of thalidomide.

Studies of nutritional support, including enteral and parenteral feeding, generally have shown no significant improvement in patient survival or tumour shrinkage and only limited effects on the complications associated with surgery, radiotherapy and chemotherapy (Klein & Koretz, 1994). Unfortunately most of the studies in this area have not measured the impact of nutritional support on symptoms and performance status in advanced cancer. In a study of Bennegard *et al.* (1983) weight losing patients treated with tube feedings for two weeks showed a significant increase in weight and body cell mass, despite a significant decrease in spontaneous food intake. However, a drawback to enteral tube feeding remains the considerable distress to patients in the case of long-term treatments (Laviano & Meguid, 1996). Enteral feeding has also been associated with significant morbidity in some cases – mainly due to aspiration, pneumonia and diarrhoea (Bruera & Fainsinger, in Doyle *et al.*, 1998).

In case of total parenteral nutrition (TPN), efficacy has not been proven and its use is not recommended in view of this and the practical disadvantages and increased risk of complications (Simons, 1997).

Aggressive nutritional therapy does not seem to influence the outcome of patients with advanced cancer. Nonetheless its use could be warranted in some conditions, such as when patients are recovering from surgery and awaiting chemotherapy, or when starvation in patients with extremely slow-growing tumours or bowel obstruction is caused by lack of food rather than metabolic abnormalities (Laviagno & Meguid, 1996; Bruera & Neumann, 1998).

Future studies on anorexia should focus on the interaction between several symptoms, like cachexia, chronic nausea, pain, asthenia, anorexia, depression and anxiety. Symptomatic benefit should be considered as the main outcome in studies in which the effects of nutritional and pharmacological interventions are tested in randomised trials.

7.8   Assessment and management of constipation

Constipation is a frequent and disabling symptom in terminally ill patients. It may be associated with abdominal pain and distension, nausea and vomiting, urinary retention and cognitive impairment, contributing to further decline in the quality of life of patients. Constipation may develop from different causes, such as mechanical obstruction, metabolic disturbances, neurological disorders, advanced age, confusion, sedation, reduced physical activity, low fluid intake and depression, but the use of opioids is one of the main causes in this population. Effective treatment of constipation starts with a careful assessment, including the history and frequency and difficulty of defecation, symptoms caused by constipation, and physical and rectal examination. When the diagnosis of constipation is unclear, an abdominal X-ray may be required (Mancini & Bruera, 1998).

However, there is evidence that physicians and nurses (Bruera *et al.*, 1994b) frequently neglect the assessment and management of this symptom. There are no valid clinical assessment tools for constipation and future studies should focus on developing measurement instruments, including self-assessment tools for patients and their families (Mancini & Bruera, 1998).

Despite prophylaxis, a majority of patients with advanced disease require laxatives, but there is surprisingly little experimental evidence available to guide choice of laxative type and dosage (Sykes in Doyle *et al.*, 1998). Therapeutic interventions for the routine management of constipation may be administered orally or rectally. Oral laxatives include bulk agents, osmotic agents, contact cathartics, and agents for colonic lavage, lubricants, prokinetic drugs and oral naloxone (Mancini & Bruera, 1998). Lactulose and senna are the most popular laxatives in hospice care and the two drugs are often used in combination because of the stool-softening effect of lactulose and the relatively greater peristalsis-stimulating effect of senna. Promising drugs seem to be naloxone and cisapride. Naloxone has shown success experimentally in patients receiving strong opioid analgesia (Sykes, 1991; Culpepper-Morgan *et al.*, 1992; Sykes, 1996). A prokinetic agent, cisapride appears to hold considerable promise for patients suffering from colonic and intestinal motility disorders. Future research is needed to clarify the role of this agent in opioid-induced constipation (McCalum, 1991; Barone *et al.*, 1994; Sykes in Doyle *et al.*, 1998; Mancini & Bruera, 1998).

For acute short-term management and severe episodes of constipation, enemas and rectal suppositories may be used. Occasional patients who cannot tolerate oral laxatives may be able to use long-term rectal laxatives or enemas effectively. Rectal laxatives may be lubricant, osmotic, surfactant, aline or polyphenolic. If concurrent usage of rectal laxative measures is an indication of the ineffectiveness of oral laxatives, results of oral laxatives seem poor. Between 40% and 57% of hospice patients receive rectal measures on a continuing basis (Sykes in Doyle *et al.*, 1998).

There is much scope for further work on the comparative efficacy of laxatives. Randomised clinical trials comparing different laxatives are badly needed. One of the main limitations of such a trial is the lack of a reliable and valid clinical assessment tool.

7.9 Assessment and management of depression

Terminally ill patients are particularly vulnerable to depression. The incidence increases with higher levels of disability, pain and advanced illness. Approximately 25% of all cancer patients experience severe depressive symptoms and among patients with advanced illness 77% is mentioned (Bukberg *et al.*, 1984). Payne (1998) reported, based on a review of 12 articles between 1992 and 1996, depression rates ranging from 3% to 69%. Certain types of cancer are associated with an increased incidence of depression (Breitbart in Doyle *et al.*, 1998). For example, patients with pancreatic cancer are more likely to develop depression than patients with other types of intra-abdominal malignancies (Alter, 1996). In a study of Chochinov *et al.* (1994) 9% of terminally ill patients met the criteria for a major depression. Psychiatric disorders in another study of patients with pain were adjustment disorder with depressed mood (69%) and major depression (15%) (Breitbart in Doyle *et al.*, 1998).

Depressed mood can be an appropriate response to illness and grief over the impending loss of one's life, loved ones and autonomy. Kuuppelomaki & Lauri (1998), who conducted a study on cancer patients' reported experiences of suffering, concluded that the negative changes in the body, the pain, dependence, helplessness and inability to do anything caused psychological distress and depression. Depression found expression in a sense of being shocked or feeling weak, apathetic and paralysed. Other possible causes or risk factors for depression might be changes in relationships, practical issues such as finance and lack of support from family and friends (Barraclough, 1997).

It is important to recognise psychiatric disorders because, if untreated, they add to patients' suffering. Various misconceptions about psychiatric disorders in medical patients contribute to the widespread under-recognition and under-treatment of depression. The diagnosis of a major depression in terminally ill patients relies more on the psychological or cognitive symptoms of major depression than the somatic signs and symptoms (Massie & Holland, 1990). The presence of fatigue, change in appetite and loss of energy is often not helpful in establishing a diagnosis of depression in this population because terminal illness itself can produce many of these physical symptoms so characteristic of major depression.

For this reason, several efforts have been made to develop screening inventories. One of the most widely used instruments in sick populations is the hospital anxiety and depression scale (HADS) (Zigmond & Snaith, 1983). It is used widely in cancer patients but its application in palliative care is still to be tested (Doyle *et al.*, 1998). In the review article of Payne (1998) the HADS was used by Payne (1992), Spiller and Alexander (1993) and Maher *et al.* (1996). Other studies used the general health questionnaire (GHQ) (Kaasa *et al.*, 1993) or the mood evaluation questionnaire (Melvin *et al.*, 1995). The HADS was the most frequently used measure as it discriminates between depression and anxiety and excludes somatic symptoms which may be confounded with the disease process (Payne, 1998).

Le Fevre and others (1999) performed a comparison study between the HADS and the GHQ in a palliative care setting. They concluded that the HADS appears to be an effective screening instrument for psychiatric illness, particularly depression, in the palliative care inpatient setting and outperforms the GHQ. However, some critical notes were made by Payne (1998) who stated that the use of the HADs might be problematic in palliative care as it contains statements that may be inappropriate in this patient group.

Chochinov *et al.* (1997) compared the performance of four brief screening measures for depression in a group of terminally ill patients. Semistructured diagnostic interviews for depression were administered to 197 patients receiving palliative care. The interview served as the standard against which the screening performance of the four brief screening methods was assessed. He found that a single-item interview screening correctly identified the eventual diagnostic outcome of every patient, substantially outperforming the questionnaire (Beck depression inventory) and visual analogue measures.

Depression among patients with advanced disease can be managed by utilising a combination of anti-depressant medications, supportive counselling and cognitive-behavioural techniques.

Psychotherapeutic interventions have been shown to be effective in reducing depressive symptoms in cancer patients, either in individual or group sessions (Spiegel *et al.*, 1981; Spiegel & Bloom, 1983; Massie *et al.*, 1989). Holland *et al.* (1988) provided evidence of the effectiveness of behavioural techniques, such as relaxation and distraction. Although these kinds of therapies have proven to be effective, pharmacotherapy is the mainstay for treating depression of terminally ill patients (Doyle *et al.*, 1998). The prognosis and the time frame for treatment play an important role in determining the type of pharmacotherapy. Three groups of antidepressants can be considered for use in cancer patients:

(1) Newer antidepressants, including selective serotonin re-uptake inhibitors (SSRIs) and reversible inhibitors of the monoamine oxidase
(2) Tricyclic antidepressants
(3) Psychostimulants.

(Bruera & Neumann, 1998)

There is little information available on the prescribing and effectiveness of antidepressant medication in terminally ill patients but there is some evidence for under-treatment. Goldberg *et al.* (1986) studied the use of psychotropics in 202 terminally ill patients and found that 6% were prescribed antidepressants within the final six weeks of life and 3% within the final week of life.

Stiefel *et al.* (1990) found in a study about changes in psychotropic prescribing in the USA that antidepressants were underused. Lloyd-Williams *et al.* (1999) reviewed 1046 patient admissions. It appears from this study that only a few patients receiving hospice-based palliative care were prescribed antidepressant medication and that in the majority of cases medication was given so late that there was insufficient time for a response prior to death. Patients prescribed antidepressants were significantly younger than those who were not and patients with breast cancer were prescribed antidepressant medication more frequently than other patient groups. There were no prescriptions for psychostimulants. It can be concluded that there appears to be a need for research in both the assessment and treatment of depression in terminally ill patients.

7.10 Assessment and management of delirium

Delirium is common among patients with advanced disease. The prevalence of delirium in cancer patients is estimated to range from 20% in hospitalised or ambulatory patients to as high as 75% in terminally ill cancer patients. Delirium has been defined as an etiologically, non-specific, global, cerebral dysfunction characterised by concurrent disturbances of level of consciousness, attention, thinking, perception, memory, psychomotor behaviour, emotion and the sleep-wake cycle (Breitbart & Jacobsen, 1996). Delirium is conceptualised as a reversible process; however it may not be reversible in the last two days of life. This is due to the fact that irreversible processes such as multiple organ failure are occurring.

The causes of delirium in palliative care patients may vary. Although delirium may occasionally be due to the direct effect of cancer on the central nervous system (primary brain tumour or cerebral, leptomeningeal metastases), delirium is more often related to the indirect effects of cancer like metabolic changes due to organ failure, treatment side effects from medication, infection, haematologic abnormalities, changes in electrolyte balance and nutrition (Roth and Breitbart, 1996). Patients with pain and other severe symptoms are more likely to develop major psychiatric complications like confusion or depression (Derogatis *et al.*, 1983; Glover *et al.*, 1995; Roth & Breitbart, 1996).

Due to the fragile physiological state of terminally ill patients a large number of medications may engender an episode of delirium. Certainly opioid analgesics play an important role in the development of confusional states. Minagawa *et al.* (1996) studied 93 terminally ill patients who were systematically assessed for psychiatric disorders using the minimal mental state examination and structured clinical interview for classification system DSM 3 within one week of admission to a palliative care unit in a hospital. In 28% of the subjects delirium was observed. Patients with delirium had a worse prognosis and greater impairment in Karnofsky performance status. It was also noted that patients with delirium suffered significantly higher mortality than control populations. The ability to predict life expectancy of patients with advanced cancer has been poor even among experienced clinicians. Thus, the presence of delirium may be helpful in predicting the life expectancy of patients who receive palliative care (Minagawa *et al.*, 1996).

Mercadante *et al.* (1997) performed a longitudinal survey using 325 cancer patients. All were advanced cancer patients with pain that required opioid therapy for more than six weeks before death. An opioid escalation index was used to index the mean increase of the starting dosage, expressed as a percentage or in mg. The authors found that an increase of this index was associated with the presence of confusion. Moreover the presence of confusion was associated with neuropathic pain.

Widely used instruments to facilitate the diagnosis of delirium are the minimal mental state examination (Folstein *et al.* 1975) and the delirium rating scale (Trzepacz *et al.*, 1988). The minimal mental state examination involves a series of questions and tasks that assess orientation, registration, attention and calculation, recall and language. The delirium rating scale is a 10-item clinician-rated scale and is able to distinguish delirium from other neuropsychiatric disorders.

Management of delirium in the terminally ill involves treatment of the underlying cause if possible, eliminating non essential drugs that can worsen confusion, environmental manipulations and the use of antipsychotic drugs to control symptoms and agitated behaviour, and attempt to clear the patient's sensorium (Passik & Cooper, 1999). A common approach to management of confusion caused by opioid therapy is to lower the dose if the pain is under control or to change to another opioid (Roth & Breitbart, 1996).

Symptomatic and supportive therapies are important as well (Breitbart & Jacobsen, 1996). Fluid and electrolyte balance, nutrition and vitamins, as well as a quiet well-lit room with familiar objects and the presence of family or nurse, may be helpful. Roth and Breitbart (1996) also suggest that frequent reminders by staff or family of location, day, time and outside events help distract patients from their internal thoughts, hallucinations or delusions and afford them appropriate orientation.

Neuroleptics and benzodiazepines are found to be useful in the management of delirium. The majority of delirious patients can be effectively treated with oral haloperidol. In order to sedate the agitated delirious patients, lorazepam along with haloperidol may be effective (Roth & Breitbart, 1996). Midazolam and methotrimeprazine are also used to sedate. Passik and Cooper (1999) suggest that newer atypical antipsychotics have potential for the treatment of delirium and also have the added benefit of causing less akathisia and other extrapyramidal side effects. Olanzapine may be a useful agent for the oncology population. Conceivably its activity at multiple types of receptors may translate into utility in a number of psychiatric and other syndromes. The role of these atypical antipsychotics in the treatment of delirium needs to be further investigated in formal trials.

7.11 Conclusions

In this chapter an overview has been given of the symptoms most prevalent in palliative care. A number of symptoms have been found to be more prevalent than others. All symptoms nevertheless, irrespective of their prevalence, seem to impact on the terminally ill patients' daily functioning and quality of life. In addition to citing the symptom prevalence in adults with terminal illness, attention has been given where possible to management techniques in symptom relief.

As mentioned earlier, in the introduction, this chapter is not intended to be exhaustive in nature but rather exemplary. A review of the state of the art with regard to symptom assessment and management is a topic of its own and as such deserves more attention in future research. Future research should focus on the development of measurement instruments in order to measure the prevalence of symptoms or to be used as outcome measure in clinical trials. A growing need is evident for randomised clinical trials that can prove the efficacy of treatment. More attention is also warranted for methodological problems in measuring symptoms. Randomised clinical trials are seldom used in terminally ill patients due to the methodological and ethical dilemmas they pose. Researchers in this area are advised to focus on some of these issues. Little is known in addition about the actual management of symptoms by clinicians; how clinical decisions and diagnoses are made and how symptoms are managed in the practice setting are important research topics and warrant attention in the future.

Chapter 8

Pain and Symptom Management in Children

Huda Huijer Abu-Saad

8.1 Introduction

Pain and symptom management continue to be cited as challenges for health professionals and lay caregivers in paediatric palliative care. Fears of promoting addiction, tolerance and physical dependence are being replaced by ethical questions and concerns that aggressive pain management may be a form of euthanasia. The art and science of pain control in the terminally ill child witnessed a major transformation in the 1990s. Physicians and nurses in this field have an obligation to remain up-to-date and to seek consultation from pain specialists if the situation arises and when reasonable patient comfort has not been achieved. Patients with metastasis to spine and major nerves may require extraordinary measures including epidural and subarachnoid infusions to achieve adequate analgesia.

8.2 Symptom prevalence

In a retrospective survey over a five-year period of the signs and symptoms encountered by children during the last months of life, Hunt (1990) reported pain, sweating, psychological distress, seizures, cough and swallowing difficulty to be the symptoms most persistent. In the last week of life, however, muscle spasms, excess secretions, dyspnoea, seizures, oral symptoms, pain and cough were found to be most prevalent. The symptoms found most difficult to control were muscle spasm and excessive secretions. In another study looking at the medical and nursing problems encountered by children with neurodegenerative disease admitted to a hospice for children, Hunt and Burne (1995) found that the majority of the children had died at home.

Examination of the most commonly encountered problems revealed that nearly all the children had no speech or speech was impaired, and most children were totally immobile or had reduced mobility. In addition, the majority of the children had feeding problems and were fed through a nasogastric tube or gastrostomy. These children were also found to have suffered occasional pain, with muscle spasm being the main identifiable source of pain. In a study of children enrolled in a palliative care programme in the terminal phase of the disease, Humbert (1997) found that up to 90% had pain, 35% nausea and vomiting, 35% dyspnoea, and 25% convulsions.

Pain in a child with cancer poses a significant challenge for health professionals. A number of studies addressed the prevalence and nature of pain in paediatric and young adult patients with cancer. Cornaglia *et al.* (1984), in a retrospective chart review study, reported that 57% of children with cancer had pain of moderate or severe intensity. Miser *et al.* (1987a,b) found pain to be the most frequently presenting symptom of patients treated at the paediatric branch of the National Cancer Institute in the USA. A large number of these patients reported having moderate to severe pain. The predominant cause of pain for the majority of patients was found to be treatment-related and included mucositis, neuropathies, phantom limb and infections. Tumour-related pain accounted for the discomfort experienced by one-third of the patients and was mostly prevalent in patients with active disease and metastatic bone disease. In a study conducted by Elliott *et al.* (1991) on the epidemiological features of pain in pediatric cancer patients, 58% of the pain was found to be related to the side-effects of anti-cancer treatment, 21% was related to the cancer itself, and 21% was non-cancer related. The predominance of treatment-related rather than cancer-related pain differs from results found among adult cancer patients.

8.3   Pain and symptom management

Almost all children with cancer and other terminal diseases will experience pain during the course of their illness. This can be related to the disease itself, to the effects of the therapy instituted, to invasive procedures, and to the multitude of psychological factors associated with the child's condition. Pain control in children with cancer and for all children receiving palliative care should include regular pain assessments, appropriate analgesics administered at regular dosing intervals, adjunctive drug therapy for symptom and side effects control, and non-pharmacological interventions to modify the situational factors that can exacerbate the child's pain and suffering. These reasons among others have led to the development of the WHO guidelines on cancer pain relief and palliative care in children, and to this issue becoming a major priority in a comprehensive WHO cancer programme (McGrath, P.A., 1996).

Pain assessment

A number of factors should be taken into consideration when assessing chronic pain in children with cancer and in terminally ill children in general (see Fig. 8.1). The conceptual model for chronic pain in children depicts the inter-relatedness of a number of factors and their impact on the quality of life of the child in pain. These include physical, psychological, social, cultural and spiritual as well as demographic variables. For further information the reader is referred to Abu-Saad (1993).

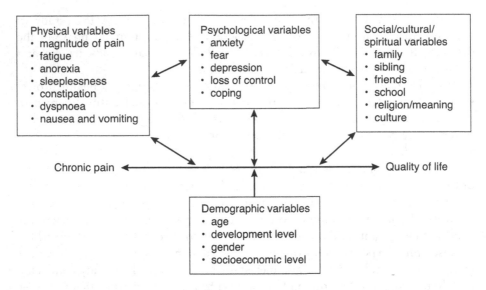

Fig. 8.1 Conceptual model for chronic pain in children.

Effective symptom management necessitates frequent and regular assessment, taking into consideration the viewpoints of the child and parents. The care plan needs to include regular monitoring of the pain using an assessment tool appropriate for the child's developmental level. A number of pain assessment tools have been developed and validated for use with children. The appropriateness of these tools for the terminally ill child, however, has never been investigated and deserves as a result more attention in the future. Of particular importance is the development of a tool that is simple to understand and easy to use by both children and parents. The principle remains that children should become as involved as possible in their own care, depending on their age and level of understanding. For preverbal children and those unable to communicate because of developmental delays or multiple handicaps, assessments of pain must rely on the primary caretakers who are usually the parents. For some young children assessment may involve using a simple tool at the bedside (Arts *et al.*, 1994). For older children and adolescents, keeping a personal journal with records of the level of pain and the effects of treatment and symptom control will provide them with a sense of self-control over their pain and ultimately over the care provided.

The most valuable information about children's pain is obtained by assessing their subjective pain experience. Using the right methods, children as young as three years can provide adequate information on their pain experience. Multidimensional pain questionnaires are available which address the intensity, frequency, duration, quality, effect, coping strategies and impact of the pain on daily activities. These include the Abu-Saad pediatric pain assessment tool (PPAT) (Abu-Saad, 1989, 1994; Abu-Saad *et al.*, 1990, 1994; Abu-Saad & Uiterwijk, 1995), the Varni-Thompson pediatric pain questionnaire (VTPPQ)

(Varni *et al.*, 1987), the children's comprehensive pain questionnaire (CCPQ) (McGrath, 1998), and the Gustave Roussy pain scale (Douleur Enfant Gustave Roussy (DEGR)) (Gauvain-Piquard *et al.*, 1999).

The PPAT (see Table 8.1) assesses present and worst pain intensity using a 10 cm scale, pain quality using 30 word descriptors of pain, as well as pain coping and impact of pain on daily activities. The tool has been validated for use in children with cancer. In addition, a multitude of measures for assessing pain intensity is also available. These include visual analogue scales and their variations (Abu-Saad, 1984, 1994; Abu-Saad *et al.*, 1990, 1994; Abu-Saad & Uiterwijk, 1995) (see Fig. 8.2), Faces pain scales (Bieri *et al.*, 1990) (see Fig. 8.3), and the use of photographs such as the Oucher scale (Beyer & Aradine, 1984) (see Fig. 8.4). For more information on pain scales see Finley and McGrath (1998). Detailed information on a child's pain is important for an accurate diagnosis and is essential in developing and evaluating an effective plan for managing pain. For an overview of pain assessment methods by age see Table 8.2.

Pain management

According to the WHO (1998) guidelines on cancer pain relief and palliative care in children, children may deny their pain for fear of more painful treatments, especially invasive procedures that appear painful to them. Parents on the other hand may not ask for aggressive pain treatments due to exaggerated fears of drug addiction and misunderstandings about how drugs work. Among health professionals a number of barriers to proper pain control have also been identified:

- Unfounded fear of addiction can lead physicians to administer opioid analgesics as a last resort. Children may not receive as a result the most potent analgesics to relieve severe cancer pain.
- Misunderstandings over the pharmacokinetics of opioids in children may lead to the use of inadequate doses, given at inappropriate intervals, and by unnecessarily painful or less effective routes.
- Lack of knowledge about the nature of children's perception of pain and illness, which leads to inadequate evaluation of all the factors contributing to pain, may result in inadequate treatment.
- Lack of information about the simple behavioural, cognitive and supportive techniques to reduce pain.

Palliative care for children dying of cancer, according to the WHO (1998) guidelines, should be part of a comprehensive approach that addresses their physical symptoms, and their psychological, cultural and spiritual needs. It should be possible to provide such care in the child's home if the child and family so wish.

According to the WHO guidelines the four key concepts underlying the effective management of pain are: 'by the ladder', 'by the clock', 'by the mouth',

Table 8.1 The Abu-Saad Pediatric Pain Assessment Tool (PPAT) – quality and intensity of pain.

Word descriptors of pain		
Sensory	Affective	Evaluative
burning	sad	unbearable
shooting	fearful	miserable
cutting	sickening	horrible
stinging	tiring	uncomfortable
sharp	cruel	
drilling	punishing	
cramping	whining	
pumping		
hurting		
like needles		
beating		
pricking		
pinching		
tingling		
pulling		
pounding		
squeezing		
itching		
throbbing		

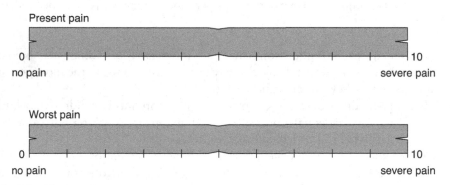

Fig. 8.2 10 cm scale.

and 'by the child'. 'By the ladder' refers to the three-step approach for selecting progressively stronger analgesics – acetaminophen, codeine, and morphine – based on the child's pain level: mild, moderate and strong. 'By the clock' refers to the timing of administration. Analgesics should be administered on a regular basis based on the drugs' duration of action and the child's pain severity and not on a PRN basis. 'By the mouth' refers to the route of drug administration. Medications should be administered to children by the simplest effective route, which in this case is the mouth. Since children may be scared of injections, they may deny having pain in order to avoid receiving an injection. This may lead to

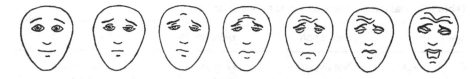

Fig. 8.3 Faces pain scale (Finley & McGrath, 1998).

undertreatment of pain. 'By the child' means that medications given to children should be based on each child's individual circumstances. There is no single medication and no one defined dose that is appropriate for all children with pain.

Many children with life-threatening diseases need opioid medication for pain

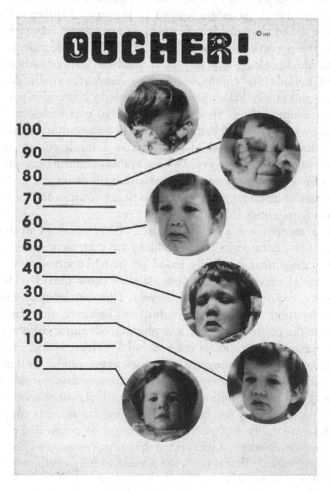

Fig. 8.4 Oucher pain scale (Finley & McGrath, 1998).

Table 8.2   Pain assessment methods by age in children.

Age	Self-report	Behavioural	Physiological
Birth to 3 years	Not available	Of primary importance	Of secondary importance
3–6 years	Possible	Of primary importance if self-report not available	Of secondary importance
Over 6 years	Of primary importance	Of secondary importance	

relief, yet there is a failure to use these medications adequately. These failures are related to misconceptions held by professionals, parents and the children them- selves. Two professional biases are known to prevent adequate use of opioid medication: the denial that children in given circumstances have pain and the diminution of the potential impact of pain. In the last case, pain is seen as a transient event with little long-term impact. In addition, fears of addiction and the side effects of opioids are common and have been repeatedly documented. Finally, patient and family biases play a major role in ineffective pain manage- ment. In some families pain is viewed as an essential part of life and is deeply rooted in their own religion and culture. Parents in some cultures tend to believe that pain will toughen up the child who can as a result endure more pain. Adolescents are known as well to avoid taking opioids because of misinformation usually propagated by schools and the media that all drugs are bad. Unfortu- nately these negative attitudes may transfer to negative attitudes for medication use and especially narcotics (McGrath, P.J., 1996).

Although oral morphine is a well-recognised opioid analgesic in the manage- ment of cancer pain, data on its use in children are extremely sparse. As a con- sequence the management is usually based on poorly controlled studies, case reports and clinical experience. In adults, studies show that a wide range of morphine doses is required to achieve analgesia. This variability among patients is not fully understood. There is some indication, however, that this difference can be related to the pharmacokinetic and pharmacodynamic differences found, and to the progression of the disease itself (Babul & Darke, 1993). Children with progressive cancer require a strong analgesic such as morphine. Oral morphine is considered the agent of first preference. Parenteral morphine should be reserved for children with recurrent vomiting and gastrointestinal disturbances. Morphine should be administered on a regular basis to achieve continuous suppression of pain. With the availability and potential usefulness of controlled-release mor- phine preparations in children, it is expected that more research will be stimulated in this area. Randomised clinical trials are needed to fully evaluate the pharma- cokinetics, dose equivalence and clinical efficacy of morphine. This will help improve pain management in terminally ill children.

To that effect and in a recent study published by Hunt *et al.* (1999) the pharmacokinetics of morphine, morphine-6-glucoronide (M6G), and morphine-3-glucuronide (M3G) were studied in children with cancer receiving morphine as immediate-release morphine liquid or sustained-release tablets. Results showed significant pharmacokinetic differences between child and adult cancer populations. Children under 11 years of age had significantly lower plasma morphine concentrations and higher morphine clearance than older children. This tendency for decreasing morphine clearance per age is similar to results found in sickle cell diseases in children. The study supports a starting dose of 1.5–2.0 mg/kg/d morphine for cancer pain unrelieved by mild to moderate strength analgesia.

In a retrospective chart review conducted by Sirkia *et al.* (1998) at the Children's Hospital in Helsinki to evaluate the need and adequacy of pain medication during terminal care of children with cancer, 89% of the children were found to have received regular pain medication. The mean duration of medication administration ranged between 17 days in children with leukaemia, 58 days in those with solid tumours, and 66 days in children with brain tumours. Anti-inflammatory drugs were first given, followed by oral morphine if deemed necessary, and finally parenteral morphine. Of the children receiving pain medication, 61% had adequate analgesia. In 19% of the children analgesia was found however, to be suboptimal. Burne and Hunt (1987), in their article describing the use of opiates in terminally ill children in the UK, found morphine and diamorphine to be commonly used in a paediatric hospice setting. Routine use of these opiates on a regular basis proved in general to be satisfactory. In some cases controlled-release morphine was helpful where analgesic requirements were stable and tablets could be given.

Goldman (1990) reported in an article on the teams' experience with controlled-release morphine (MST) given as analgesia to 60 terminally ill children with a wide range of malignant diseases. MST was found to be a useful, effective and acceptable strong analgesic for children with cancer. High doses were required and found to be tolerated by some children, particularly those with solid tumours and protracted illness. MST was given over periods ranging between 1 and 165 days. A short-acting opioid was found to be essential for breakthrough pains. Main side effects were temporary drowsiness and constipation. MST is particularly convenient for terminally ill children cared for by their parents at home. However, adequate education and supervision of its use in the home setting are, according to the author, essential.

Of particular importance in managing pain in terminally ill children is the use of the analgesic ladder recommended by WHO (Fig. 7.1). According to the ladder, if the oral route is not available an alternative route is needed. Although the transdermal administration may be a useful method for administering morphine to children, very little information is available on its usability. Collins *et al.* (1999) in a recently published article studied the feasibility, tolerability and pharmacokinetics of the therapeutic transdermal fentanyl system (TTS-fentanyl) in children with cancer pain. Results supported the feasibility and tolerability of

Table 8.3 Routes of drug administration (WHO 1998)

Oral	Transdermal	Intravenous	Subcutaneous	Intramuscular	Rectal
Painless	Painless	Rapid pain control	Avoids need for IV line	Painful	Generally disliked by
Preferred by children	Restricted to fentanyl:	Easiest to titrate and to	Useful for home	Not recommended	children
	contraindicated in	adjust to rapidly	setting	Wide variability in	Wide variability in
	opioid-naive	changing pain levels	Useful for continuous	therapeutic blood	therapeutic blood
	patients	Useful for intermittent	infusion	levels	levels
	Not indicated for acute	bolus and	Appropriate for PCA*		Variable absorption
	pain management	continuous infusion			Can be used if there is
	Not indicated for	Appropriate for PCA*			transient vomiting
	escalating pain				
	Can be used if pain				
	has been stabilised				

* PCA = patient-controlled analgesia

this method in children. In addition, results yielded pharmacokinetic parameter estimates similar to those for adults. The authors warn, however, that supplemental and rescue doses may be needed to treat breakthrough pains in this patient population.

Relieving intractable pain – pain not relieved by conventional measures – in a dying child is an extremely important aspect of palliative care. A retrospective study by Collins *et al.* (1995) performed at the Children's Hospital in Boston examined pain and opioid requirements of 199 children with terminal malignancy. The WHO analgesic ladder was the basis for the prescription of analgesics during the study period. Twelve patients (6%) were found to have intractable pain and required treatments beyond conventional opioid pharmacotherapy, eight of them requiring epidural and subarachnoid infusions and sedation to achieve adequate analgesia. The need for massive opioid treatment was found to be related to tumour spread to the spinal nerve roots, nerve plexus, and due to spinal cord compression. The authors concluded that standard dosing of opioids does adequately treat most cancer pain in children. A significant group of children nevertheless require more extensive and invasive pain management. These problems were found to occur more commonly among children with solid tumours with metastasis to spine and major nerves.

At the end of the intractable spectrum, symptoms become, however, refractory if they cannot be adequately controlled despite aggressive efforts, including those beyond conventional practice. In such a case, relief may only be possible with a therapy that compromises consciousness. Competency in treating intractable pain is thus important, not only from a humanitarian point of view, but also because the treatment of physical symptoms is a prerequisite for an adequate treatment of spiritual and psychological suffering. The memories of the dying child's parents and siblings should be that of maximal comfort in the last phase of the illness. This can only be achieved if physical distress and suffering are to a large extent minimised (Collins, 1996).

Kohler & Radford (1985) interviewed parents of 18 children who died of cancer at approximately 6 years of age. Related questionnaires were also completed. Six children experienced pain, which was subsequently controlled by adjusting oral medication. In addition to oral analgesics, local nerve blocks and diamorphine syrup were included in pain treatment.

In addition to pharmacologic pain management, numerous studies over the last two decades have demonstrated the efficacy of cognitive behavioural therapy (CBT) interventions in decreasing pain and distress in children with cancer. These strategies include simple educational preparation, systematic desensitisation, positive incentive techniques, imagery, distraction, hypnosis, relaxation and breathing strategies. Modelling and rehearsals are key components for teaching and reinforcing coping before and during procedures. Modelling involves showing the patient a video of a child the same age undergoing the same procedure, while rehearsals involve encouraging the child to practise the method with 'pretend' staff (Conte *et al.*, 1999). In recent studies, it was shown that health professionals could be taught to use these techniques and apply them in clinical settings, thus reducing the need for individuals with advanced training in this field. The use of cognitive-behavioural strategies in children with advanced cancer may have a number of advantages: children are given a sense of mastery over a stressful situation and parents are given specific roles to assist their children which may be gratifying for both. These strategies do not provide, however, a panacea and one does not have to choose between pharmacological and psychological strategies. Combinations of therapies tailored to the needs of the child and family are to be preferred and in this respect are of paramount importance.

Among the methods cited above, the use of hypnosis has been found to be effective in terminally ill children. Ellenberg *et al.* (1980) reported on using hypnosis with an adolescent girl with chronic myelogenous leukaemia during the last four months of her life. Before and after hypnosis data were collected on acute pain and anxiety during bone marrow aspiration, headache and backache, nausea and vomiting during chemotherapy, anorexia and discomfort associated with high temperatures. Hypnosis was found to be effective in reducing acute and chronic pain, anxiety and unpleasant body sensations, and partially effective in reducing nausea and vomiting.

In addition to cognitive-behavioural strategies, the WHO guidelines (1998) advocate the use of supportive and physical strategies in pain relief (see Table 8.4). Supportive therapies are intended to promote psychosocial care of children through family-centred care. To that effect, parental involvement in decision-making and in providing comfort to children is particularly important. Family-centred care encourages families to be actively involved in the care of their child, provides them with culturally appropriate information, and teaches them coping strategies. Throughout the world, culturally specific pain-reduction techniques and folk remedies are used and reflect the traditional wisdom, loyalties and trust of the family, and the social sanctions of the community. These practices must be respected and their compatibility with treatment must be established. Supporting the family involves, in addition, the provision of adequate and timely information on the diagnosis, on the illness trajectory, and on the eventual prognosis. Children must be prepared according to their age and developmental level and more importantly should never be lied to about painful procedures. They should be given the choice about the techniques that can be used in controlling pain.

Physical therapies are just as important in relieving pain. Touch is important to all children, particularly the pre-verbal child and the cognitively impaired child who understand the world to a large extent through touching and feeling. Touching includes stroking, holding and rocking, caressing, and massaging hands, feet, back, head and stomach, as well as swaddling. Touch can be the best form of communication when talking is too much of an effort for the child. In addition to touch, sources of heat and cold could be comforting for the child but should be avoided with infants because of the risk of injury. Finally transcutaneous nerve stimulation has been shown to be effective and simple to use in children, and children and families can be instructed to use the technique at home (WHO, 1998).

In summary and in order to manage pain effectively in terminally ill children, WHO (1998) recommends the use of the guidelines listed in Fig. 8.5.

Table 8.4 Non-drug methods of pain relief (WHO, 1998).

Supportive	Cognitive	Behavioural	Physical
family-centred	distraction	deep breathing	touch
Information	music	relaxation	heat and cold
empathy	imagery		TENS
choices	hypnosis		
play			

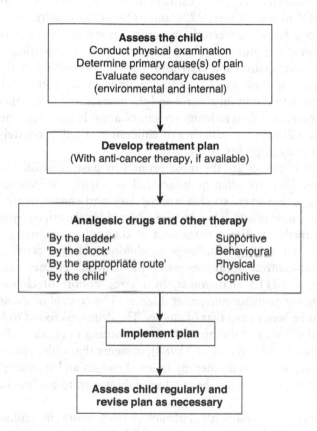

Fig. 8.5 Guidelines for pain relief in childhood cancer (WHO 1998)

Symptom management

With the exception of some studies on pain, many of the symptoms that children suffer and the approaches to relieving them have not been adequately studied. For most children with cancer, the primary goal of treatment has been to achieve a cure. Considerations of toxicity of therapy, issues regarding quality of life, and growth and development are usually secondary. To that effect, aggressive developments in medical therapies have been successful, for only 25–30% of children with cancer currently die of their disease. This concerns nevertheless a large number of children, necessitating high-quality palliative care at the end of life.

Wolfe *et al.* (2000), in a study looking at symptoms and suffering at the end of life, interviewed 103 parents of children who died of cancer. Results showed that 49% of these children died in hospital and nearly half of these deaths occurred in the intensive care unit. Based on parents' reports, 89% of children were found to suffer 'a lot' and ' a great deal' from at least one symptom and 51% from three or more symptoms. Most commonly encountered symptoms were fatigue, pain and dyspnoea. Other symptoms included poor appetite, nausea and vomiting, constipation and diarrhoea. The treatment of pain and dyspnoea was found only to be successful in respectively, 27% and 16% of the children. A considerable discordance was found between the reporting of symptoms by parents and the documentation of symptoms by physicians, with parents reporting more fatigue, poor appetite, constipation and diarrhoea. Lack of recognition of the problem by the medical team in these cases may lead to unnecessary suffering by the child. Greater attention to symptom control and the overall well being of children with advanced disease, as well as to better communication between parents and health professionals, will ease the suffering of children and will ultimately lead to an improvement in their quality of life.

Nausea and vomiting are the most prominent gastrointestinal symptoms in palliative care. They are often multifactorial in origin. The predominant cause must be sought, however, so that appropriate anti-emetic treatments can be instituted. Very little research has been conducted on the effectiveness of specific management methods. The management of chemotherapy-induced emesis, for example, presents a major challenge in children. Hewitt *et al.* (1993), in a European multicentred study, assessed the clinical efficacy and safety of Ondansetron, a 5-HT3 anatagonist, in a large cohort of children receiving chemotherapy regimens for malignant diseases. The control of nausea, however, was shown to be better than that of emesis. The drug was found to be safe, well-tolerated, and effective in the prevention of vomiting in children. Based on pre-liminary studies by LeBaron *et al.* (1988), it seems that older children and girls might experience more chemotherapy-induced nausea and vomiting than infants and boys. More studies need to be conducted, however, to confirm or reject these results.

Constipation is a commonly encountered symptom in palliative care in children and is usually a side-effect of opioid therapy. Constipation should be anticipated and treated vigorously. Oral drugs are usually preferred in combination with stool softeners such as lactulose. Rectal measures may be needed if prophylaxis is unsuccessful. Simple measures to combat constipation include increasing the child's mobility and improving their diet and fluid intake.

Respiratory symptoms which may be the cause of distress for children and their parents include dyspnoea, cough and excess secretions. If the underlying cause of dyspnoea cannot be found or if it is not amenable to treatment, the best relief can be sought in combining a number of drug methods with practical and supportive approaches. The sensation of breathlessness can be decreased using opioid drugs. A sedative may also be helpful in relieving anxiety. Children with dyspnoea in the late stages of a malignant disease do not find oxygen helpful and often dislike the use of facial masks. The confidence of the staff to manage the situation, including the acute problems, is essential. Simple measures such as finding the optimum position, not crowding the room, keeping curtains and windows open, and relaxation exercises should be used according to the child's needs and what seems to be the most helpful at that particular time (Goldman, 1994).

8.4   Care of the dying child

The needs of dying children are often neglected because emotional reactions in children are typically often overlooked. A difficult issue for parents of terminally ill children is what to tell their children. Parents are known to protect their children by providing them with as little upsetting information as possible. Children on the other hand do sense the anxiety and upheaval of the parents and in order not to upset them they sometimes feign ignorance. All these factors heighten children's anxiety and isolation and leave them unsure of whom to trust. It is thus of paramount importance that parents and health professionals are as honest as possible about the diagnosis and treatment and provide adequate and appropriate information while taking into consideration the children's developmental level. Even more difficult for parents is discussing the ultimate diagnosis with children.

The ability of children to understand and recognise what death is and that death is pending, is to a great part dependent on their developmental level. Infants have no cognitive understanding of death. Pre-school-age children understand death as temporary and reversible; they are egocentric and view death as punishment or wish fulfilment, and may believe they have caused death. School-age children and pre-adolescents view death as permanent, real, final and universal but they are unable sometimes to comprehend their own mortality. Adolescents on the other hand have a good comprehension of the existential implications of death, especially as they gain more of an ability to think abstractly. They do deny, however, their own mortality through risk-taking behaviour (Barakat *et al.*, 1995). Consequently children, based on their developmental level, must be able to determine the pace at which they address the issue of death.

Of particular importance in this case is that children must lead as normal a life as possible once the crisis of initial diagnosis and treatment has passed. Over-protectiveness should be avoided as much as possible in order for children not to lose independence that is already limited by the illness itself. This means that children should resume their regular activities as much as possible; a return to school if at all possible should be attempted. Children cared for at home are entitled as a result to the provision for play and education in accordance with their developmental level and physical abilities. These provisions give the children a vital sense of normality and continuity and enable them to develop short-term goals and an essential sense of purpose in their lives (Liben, 1998). In a study conducted in France by Bouffet *et al.* (1996), school intervention programmes for children and adolescents with cancer were evaluated. Results from 30 children requiring palliative care were prospectively collected. Sixty per cent of the children showed a continuous desire for school education throughout their life's end. Reading, mathematics and computers were the favourite topics. With 40% of the children, however, the schools refused to collaborate; their refusal was related to extra-academic topics and uncontrolled pain.

Children with a terminal illness will have fears and fantasies about their illness and the impending death and they should be encouraged to express them in a setting of their choice where they feel most comfortable. Some children will show evidence of poor adjustment to death by exhibiting behaviours such as irritability, separation anxiety and clinging, fear of the dark, non-compliance, regressive behaviours, somatic complaints, sleep and eating disturbances, decreased interest in play or other activities, poor concentration and preoccupation with death. The use of imagery can provide, according to LeBaron & Zeltzer (1985), an alternative way of communication. Clinical cases, based on the authors' experience, illustrate some of the ways in which imagery may play a crucial role in helping terminally ill children to express their needs and fears regarding helplessness, separation from loved ones and death.

8.5   Conclusions

This chapter has addressed an important aspect of palliative care in children – the management of prevalent and exacerbating symptoms. Of particular importance is the management of pain and other related symptoms and the ensuing side effects. In the area of pain some strides have been made. There is a great deal to be done yet in testing the clinical utility of assessment tools, evaluating the effectiveness of pharmacological and non-pharmacological management strategies, and in addressing the issues related to the pharmacokinetics and pharmacodynamics of the majority of the drugs currently in use in palliative care. The field is still open when it comes to assessing other symptoms and testing the effectiveness of specific symptom-relieving interventions. More research work is warranted in this area.

For children, death is an abstract concept that is at times difficult to comprehend. Pain and other symptoms are, however, real; children often confuse fear of pain with the fear of death. Pain needs as a result to be adequately managed by skilled professionals and specialists with experience in pain management of the terminally ill child. Inadequate pain management related to health professionals' fears about addiction or due to lack of knowledge might have detrimental effects on the child and their family. Dealing effectively with the physical concerns of children will enable the child and the family to deal better with the psychosocial issues.

Chapter 9

Instruments to Assess Quality of Palliative Care

Annemie Courtens

9.1 Introduction

Improving quality of palliative care requires measurement tools that are valid, reliable and clinically relevant. Donabedian's (1980) model on quality indicators in health care with emphasis on structure, process and outcome is of particular relevance for palliative care research. To improve services it is necessary to pay attention to all three elements. Structure and process are important for the outcomes they produce, while outcomes can only be changed through the structures and processes that produce them. The key aspect of quality improvement, however, is measuring the outcomes of care. (Health) outcomes are being promoted as a necessary evaluation measure of care services.

Outcomes can be seen as the result of clinical interventions. They are divided into patient-centred outcomes and organisation-centred outcomes. Patient-centred outcomes include patient satisfaction with care, symptom management, functional status and quality of life. Organisation-centred outcomes focus on quality of care issues such as what staff do and how they deliver services, and how they communicate and give information and practical support, as well as data on mortality and morbidity.

This chapter addresses first the importance of the measurement of outcome variables in palliative care research. Secondly, a brief summary is given of the instruments developed and tested in this area and methodological issues are discussed. Finally, recommendations are made where improvement in instrumentation is still warranted. This chapter is not intended to be exhaustive. A review of the state of the art with regard to research on the experienced quality of life of patients and their families is a topic of its own and hence deserves more attention in future research. This is not an easy job. Differences in methodologies, patient populations and instruments make it hard to draw conclusions.

9.2   Quality of life and other outcomes in palliative care research

In palliative care it is often stated that improved quality of life is the overriding goal, the primary target for assessment and outcome to be evaluated. Although many authors have tried to define quality of life in different ways, there is consensus that the concept is a multidimensional entity and that quality of life should reflect the experience of the individual's physical, psychological, social and existential dimension and is strongly influenced by subjective factors. Brady and Cella (1999) define the subjective nature of health-related quality of life in the palliative setting as: the extent to which one's usual or expected physical, emotional, social and spiritual well being are affected by a medical condition or its treatment. They state that it is important to recognise that patients' perceptions of their illness are extremely variable and factors other than the actual disability enter into that perception. This also means that although symptoms or functional status are important components of quality of life, it is more than a simple summary of symptoms or functional status.

The last two decades of the twentieth century witnessed the emergence of quality of life as a major outcome variable in health care research. Oncology was historically one of the first medical disciplines to consider explicitly not only the clinical but also the psychosocial variables in evaluating therapeutic interventions. Not only quantity but also quality of survival has become important. The quest for quality is especially prominent in palliative care where symptom-control rather than curative interventions are of importance. Relevant questions regarding quality of life are important in palliative care and research may include:

- Describing how patients feel along the disease trajectory.
- Obtaining more information on the patients' problems and needs for better clinical monitoring.
- Evaluating which therapeutic strategies for stabilising disease and achieving symptom control are most beneficial in improving quality of life.
- Comparing the efficacy and cost-effectiveness of services in relation to maintenance and improvement of quality of life.
- Identifying the potential for enhancing patients' quality of life with new medical, nursing and paramedical interventions. As palliative care develops, the effectiveness of these newly developed interventions should be scientifically tested.
- Auditing the care provided to determine whether standards of care are being used and to identify potential areas for improvement.

In order to investigate these issues in a scientific fashion assessment of quality of life, symptoms and functional status as well as quality of care is necessary. Questionnaires that itemise likely problems can provide an efficient and systematic way to ensure that needs are addressed (Brady & Cella, 1999). Lists or instruments might be helpful, for example in fatigued and cognitively impaired patients. It is easier to identify and define their needs when possible needs are listed in front of them, rather than having to generate ideas spontaneously (Brady & Cella, 1999). Besides, these quality of life instruments can be used as a tool to facilitate communication between staff and patient.

9.3   Outcome measures: symptoms, functional status, quality of life and quality of care instruments in palliative care

A thorough review of the literature resulted in the identification of a number of instruments which are either specifically developed for health-related quality of life research in cancer or have been adapted for that purpose. Since the mid 1980s a variety of instruments have been developed but few have been designed specifically for use in palliative or terminal care, and validation of new hospice-based instruments is still very much in its infancy.

A review of the literature yielded eight measures, which satisfied the following inclusion criteria:

- Assessing more than one of the above-mentioned dimensions of palliative care (physical, psychological, social and existential)
- Targeting the population of patients with advanced disease or palliative care
- Reliable, valid and appropriate for the target population.

Most of these instruments were developed for use in clinical audits or to measure the effectiveness of care. Some of them focus on symptoms (ESAS) or functional status (EFAT) alone, while others combine symptoms, functional status, general quality of life, future placement or existential issues (PACA, MQOL, MQLS, EORTC QLQ). The STAS and POS consist of a mix of symptoms: quality of life and quality of care issues. (See the following sections for explanations of these instruments.)

The Edmonton Symptom Assessment System (ESAS)

Bruera *et al.* (1991) developed the ESAS (see Fig. 9.1) as an instrument for clinical audit. The schedule was developed for quick assessment in routine practice, in an inpatient setting. The tool consists of nine visual analogue scales, covering pain, activity, nausea, depression, anxiety, drowsiness, appetite, well being and shortness of breath. The schedule can be completed by the patients themselves or with nurse assistance in a few minutes.

Patients who are unable to respond due to cognitive failure are assessed by their nurse or a specially trained family member. The scores on each item can be recorded on a graph to visualise patterns of symptom control over time. Scores on the ESAS were found to correlate with scores on the support team assessment schedule (STAS). The inter-rater reliability of the instrument is good (Bruera *et al.*, 1991).

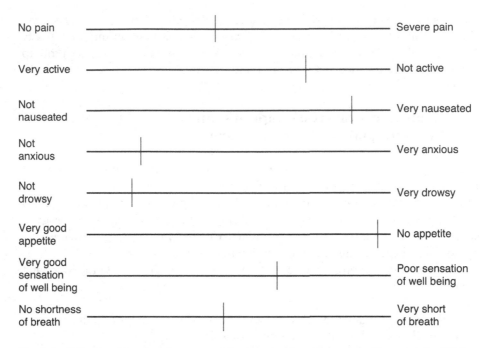

Fig. 9.1   Edmonton Symptom Assessment System visual analogue scale (Bruera et al., 1991)

The Edmonton Functional Assessment Tool (EFAT)

The EFAT was developed by Kaasa *et al*. (1997) (see Table 9.1) as a functional outcome measure for use in a palliative care population. The assessment identified ten functional activities important to patients even in the terminal stage of their illness. The inter-rater reliability, content, construct and concurrent validity have been established in a palliative population (Kaasa *et al*., 1997). The instrument consists of 11 items covering communication, mental alertness, pain, sensation, respiratory functioning, balance, mobility, activity level, wheelchair mobility, ADL and performance status. Items can be scored by patients or carers on a 4-point scale. According to Kaasa and colleagues, the EFAT was deemed to be a suitable measure of functional status in palliative care mainly because change in functioning was demonstrated over time, and repeated measures were possible without additional burden to the patient, family and team.

The Palliative Care Assessment Tool (PACA)

This instrument was developed by Ellershaw (1995) in order to assess the effectiveness of a hospital palliative care team. Symptoms like physical weakness, immobility, pain, anorexia, dry mouth, mood disturbance, anxiety, shortness of breath, constipation, loss of concentration, insomnia, nausea, vomiting, a painful mouth and diarrhoea can be scored on a 5-point scale by patients or relatives within a few minutes. Also, questions giving insight into illness and future placement are included. Insight is assessed by an observer and can be scored on a

5-point scale. Plans for the future are asked of the patient and recorded on a 4-point scale. The scores on the symptoms were found to correlate with those of the McCorcle symptom distress scale. Inter-rater reliability seems to be sufficient (Ellershaw, 1995).

The McGill Quality of Life Questionnaire (MQOL)

The MQOL developed by Cohen *et al.* (1995, 1997) is relevant to all phases of the disease trajectory for people with a life-threatening disease but has been tested in an inpatient and outpatient palliative population. The MQOL consists of 16 items and an overall QOL and open-ended question about issues that have impact on a patient's QOL. Patients are asked to report their QOL within the last two days. A rating scale from 0–10 is used.

Five domains are presented in the MQOL: physical symptoms, physical well being (e.g. physically I felt terrible – well), psychological well being (e.g. how much of the time do you feel sad, never – always), existential issues (e.g. my life to this point has been completely worthless – very worthwhile) and support (e.g. I feel close to people, completely disagree – completely agree). Patients are asked to list three problems which are perceived as the biggest problems. The acceptability, internal consistency, reliability and validity have been assessed in palliative care settings (Cohen *et al.*, 1995, 1997; Pratheepawanit *et al.*, 1999).

Construct validity of the subscales was demonstrated through correlations with the Spitzer quality of life index and the patient evaluated problem scores. Internal consistency was found to be sufficient (Pratheepawanit *et al.*, 1999). In the study of Pratheepawanit it took the patient 10–30 minutes to complete the MQOL. This was attributed mostly to the open-ended question section asking patients to describe their feelings.

The McMaster Quality of Life Scale (MQLS)

This instrument was developed by Sterkenburg *et al.* (1996) to measure quality of life in a palliative, community, inpatient or outpatient population. Thirty-two items, including physical symptoms, functional status, social functioning, emotional status, cognition, sleep and rest, energy and vitality, general life satisfaction and meaning of life, can be scored by patients, family or staff on a 7-point scale. In Sterkenburg's study, it took patients 3–30 minutes to fill in the questionnaire; staff and family took approximately three minutes.

The instrument has, according to Sterkenburg *et al.* (1996), excellent inter-rater reliability and reasonable intra-rater reliability. The overall Cronbach's alpha was high but of some subscales moderate. Systematic differences were found, depending on source of rating, suggesting that proxy rating should be avoided. The scale was shown to be sensitive to patient changes. Correlations with the Spitzer quality of life index showed evidence of concurrent validity.

Table 9.1   Edmonton functional assessment tool (Kaasa *et al.*, 1997)

	0	1	2	3
Communication	Functional Independent with all aspects of communication	Functional with assistive devices Requires glasses, hearing aids or communication devices	Moderate assist Communicates effectively <50% of time	Dependent, unable to communicate with others
Mental alert	Alert Oriented to time, place and person. Memory intact	Apathetic May be disoriented to time	Confused Intermittent to total disorientation to time place person	Unconscious Non-responsive to painful stimuli
Pain	No dysfunction Performs 75–100% of ADL/IADL Attends activities on/off unit	Minimal dysfunction Performs 50–75% of ADL/IADL without pain	Moderate dysfunction Performs 24–49% of ADL/IADL with/without rest periods because of pain	Severe dysfunction Unable to do any activities because of pain
Sensation	Intact Intact to light touch, pressure hot/cold	Minimal impairment Altered sensory impairment Limits ability to feel discomfort in one or two extremities	Severe impairment Sensory impairment Limits ability to feel discomfort in > half body surface	Absent to any of light touch, pressure, hot/cold
Respiratory function	No dysfunction	Minimal dysfunction. At least one symptom which affects patient's ability in ADL/IADL	Moderate dysfunction At least one symptom which moderately impairs patient's ability in ADL/IADL	Severe dysfunction At least one symptom which severely impairs patient's ability in ADL/IADL

Contd.

Balance	Functional Normal balance	Functional with assistance Attain/maintain position with equip one person assist	Impaired Attain/maintain position with moderate/maximal assist one or more	Absent
Mobility	Functional with/without aids Controls/moves all limbs at will	Minimal/moderate Controls/moves all limbs but degree of limitation present	Maximal assist Can assist another person who initiates Movement	Dependent Unable to assist to change position
Activity level	Functional Walks unassisted	Functional with assist Ambulate with assist of 1–2 persons/1 person and walking aid	Chairfast Ambulates only to chair with assist/confined to W/C	Bedfast Confined to bed 24 hours
Wheelchair mobility	Functional Independent in lead up and propelling	Minimal assistance Supervision with lead up/to propel	Moderate assistance Total assist with lead-up	Dependent, unable to perform
ADL	Functional Independent	Functional with adaptive devices Independent using adaptive equipment	One person assist Manual assist of one verbal cueing/supervision to complete task	Dependent total assist with ADL
Performance status	Functional Independent in room on and off unit	Minimal dysfunction Independent in room and on unit	Moderate dysfunction Assist of one in room and on unit	Severe dysfunction Assist of 1–2 persons in room

The EORTC QLQ

Another instrument that is used worldwide and has potential possibilities for use in terminal care is the EORTC QLQ-C30, a quality of life instrument for use in international clinical trials in oncology (Aaronson *et al.*, 1993). The instrument incorporates nine multi-item scales: five functional scales (physical, role, cognitive, emotional and social), three symptom scales (fatigue, pain and nausea and vomiting) and global health and quality of life scale. Several single item symptom measures are also included. Questions cover the past week and responses are mainly in the form of a 4-point Likert scale. Validity has been shown by three findings: the scores on the instrument correlated with clinical status, interscale correlations were statistically significant, and there were significant changes for patients whose performance status had improved or worsened. Internal consistency is sufficient. Patients can complete the questionnaire by themselves in approximately 11 minutes.

Kaasa *et al.* (1995) tested the list in a patient population consisting of advanced cancer patients with short life expectancy. The scale reliability was excellent for all scales, except for role functioning. The criterion validity of the emotional functioning scale was confirmed by high correlation with GHQ-20 and the pain scale was promising by correlating high with single items measuring pain frequency and intensity. A 'palliative care' module of the EORTC QLQ-C30 is currently being tested in Europe.

The Support Team Assessment Schedule (STAS)

Higginson & McCarthy (1993) developed this schedule (see Table 9.2) for use in multidisciplinary cancer support teams in community and hospice settings. It is validated to measure the effectiveness of palliative care or clinical audit. Items

Table 9.2 Items of the STAS (Higginson & McCarthy, 1993)

Pain control
Symptom control
Patient anxiety
Patient insight
Family anxiety
Family insight
Predictability
Planning
Spiritual
Communication between patient and family
Practical aid
Financial
Wasted time
Communication of professionals to patient and family
Communication between professionals
Professional anxiety
Advising professionals

---

were developed to reflect the goals of palliative care. The 17 items include pain and symptom control, insight, psychosocial, family needs, planning affairs, home service communication and support to other professionals. Patients and informal and professional caregivers (team) can fill in the STAS using a 5-point scale. The scores of professionals were found to correlate with patients' and family ratings and with other quality of life scales (Hearn & Higginson, 1997). Inter-rater reliability, internal consistency and test/retest reliability seemed to be sufficient. The instrument was shown to be valid, feasible and reliable in the Netherlands and Belgium (van den Eynden, 1994; van Cuijk, 1996; van der Steen, 1997). In very complex situations, however, it seems to be less usable.

The Palliative Care Outcome Scale (POS)

This quite new instrument was developed by Hearn and Higginson (1999) as an outcome measure for patients with advanced cancer and their families in inpatient and outpatient care, day care, home care and primary care. The POS consists of two almost identical measures, one of which is completed by staff, the other by patients. The scale was developed by using data from a review of other measures used or proposed for use in evaluating the palliative care for patients with advanced cancer. The measure consists of ten questions covering the physical, psychological and spiritual domains of quality of life in palliative care. These include pain, other symptoms, anxiety, family anxiety, information, support, life worthwhile, self worth, wasted time and personal affairs. In addition space was provided to list main problems. In a validation study (Hearn & Higginson, 1999), it took patients and staff between four and ten minutes to complete the list. The measure demonstrated construct validity (correlations with EORTC and STAS) and internal consistency. Test/retest reliability was acceptable for seven items.

9.4 Methodological issues

Development and validation of outcome measures in palliative care are still in their infancy. Methodological and practical problems regarding measuring in terminally ill patients are probably reasons for these shortcomings. In palliative care there are particular concerns about the use and relevance of outcome measures. First, patients may be very sick or in pain and thus not able to answer questions. Secondly, problems with performance status and cognitive functioning of patients may impede this process. Thirdly, patients may wish to play down symptoms to avoid expected unpleasant therapeutic repercussions or admission to hospital. Finally, some patients may clearly exaggerate problems as a legitimate way of escaping from intolerable situations (Finlay & Dunlop, 1994).

It is often assumed in 'quality of life' research that the patient's report is the gold standard. However, in the case of patients receiving palliative care there is a difficulty in using self-completion measures as many patients are too ill to complete them, or die early during care (Hearn & Higginson, 1997). This will also lead to selection bias: those patients who are likely to be experiencing the most problems are less likely to be included in data collection. For example, in the study by Byock (1994), only 45% of the people entering a hospice were able to fill in a quality of life questionnaire; the others needed some help. Mino (1999) stated that 40–70% of patients are incapable of assisting with self-assessment evaluations. This proportion increases as the disease advances.

In this patient group self-reports could be supplemented by professional or carers' reports, where appropriate, to provide the fullest picture on the patients' condition (Ahmedzai, 1990). However, there is some evidence that staff and relatives are poor estimators of patients' quality of life (Slevin *et al.*, 1988; Sprangers & Aaronson, 1992). In a study by Cohen *et al.* (1997), staff were misclassifying distressed patients as non distressed and vice versa. Grande *et al.* (1997a) found that the more a doctor perceived a symptom as being hard to control, the less frequently it was noted by that doctor. Uncontrollable symptoms were often 'missed'. Stephens *et al.* (1997) concluded from their study that doctors underestimate symptom severity 15% of the time and that there was increasing disagreement with increasing symptom severity.

In a study of Sterkenburg *et al.* (1996) it was recommended that the proxy is a relative because the correlations between relatives and patients are higher than between patients and staff. On the other hand, Higginson and McCarthy (1993) found that team ratings of the STAS were usually closer to the ratings of patients than to those of the family member. Nekolaichuk *et al.* (1999) compared patients and proxy (physician and nurse) assessments of symptoms in advanced cancer patients and concluded that average physician ratings were generally lower than patient ratings, and nurse ratings agreed more closely with patient ratings. Further research is required to map out the differences between patient and proxy ratings and the underlying reasons for the discrepancies.

Another point of discussion and of particular interest in palliative care is the difference in conceptualisation of quality of life as it applies to people who are healthy, ill or dying. There is still little known about how terminally ill patients perceive their life, what is important to them and how they weight the different components in life. In this context the so-called response-shift or positive adjustment should be mentioned: people will adjust their standard for quality of life during their illness trajectory (Sprangers & Aaronson, 1996). The purpose of many quality of life instruments is to measure improvement or deterioration in a quite stable situation. The question is whether these instruments are suitable for measurement in palliative care which is focused on the achievement of the best possible quality of life in a situation where deterioration will occur.

From the literature it is known that cancer patients reported a similar degree of life satisfaction as non-cancer patients and that non-health related domains had an increased contribution to quality of life in cancer patients (Kreitler *et al.*, 1993).

Most of the questionnaires used in 'outcome' research have been designed by professionals. They decided on the importance of concepts, items, domains and weighting, whereas a more patient-centred approach of measuring is warranted. In order for care to be successful, professionals have to understand patients' perceptions and expectations of life. If a gap exists between staff and patients' perceptions, care might not be helpful (Higginson & McCarthy, 1993).

Devery *et al.* (1999) stated in an article about health outcomes for people who use palliative care services that outcomes are perceived endpoints, and that different people may have different ideas of what these outcomes ought to be. An essential strategy in addressing this point is to ensure that all relevant parties have input in developing outcomes, including patients and informal caregivers. In other words, outcome measures and the way we obtain them should be meaningful for the patients, caregivers and other users of the services. Qualitative research methods have an important role in determining whether outcomes are meaningful. Devery *et al.* performed in-depth interviews with 77 participants about what they perceived as important in palliative care. The responses could be grouped in the following broad outcome themes: information, emotional, physical, spiritual, economic and 'multiple clients' (the involvement of family and friends). Patients and informal caregivers valued outcomes that were not necessarily brought about by expert clinical intervention. The authors suggested that by adopting too narrow interpretations of outcomes we risk sacrificing that which is uniquely valuable in palliative care services.

Quality of life instruments consequently should include those domains relevant to palliative care and in particular the physical, psychological, social and spiritual aspects of life. Most of the measures currently in use do not cover all these aspects; spirituality especially has long been neglected. Cohen *et al.* (1997) found the existential domain to be highly predictive of overall quality of life in a palliative care setting, and Brady & Cella (1999) have found a measure of spiritual well being to be as highly related to overall quality of life as is physical well being. Axelsson and Sjoden (1998) found that life meaningfulness correlated most highly with quality of life. They suggest that existential issues appear to become more important as physical status declines.

As yet, there is no golden standard for assessing outcomes in palliative care. It is advisable to choose an instrument that contributes to patient care, is brief and easy to complete, is sensitive to changes and covers important domains in palliative care, including symptoms, psychosocial concerns and spiritual and functional issues. Brady and Cella (1999) suggest that positive aspects of QOL, such as increased appreciation of life or enhanced relationships should be measured along with the negative aspects. They also consider choosing a scale that can be filled out verbally as well as in written form and avoids visual analogue scales. The VAS concept can be difficult for many palliative care patients to grasp. Numeric rating scales are probably easier to use in palliative care.

9.5 Caregiver quality of life

Several studies have documented the impact that care giving has on caregiver quality of life. Family caregivers experience increased symptoms of depression and anxiety, psychosomatic symptoms, restriction of role activities, strain in marital relationships and diminished physical health (Oberst *et al.*, 1989; Sales, 1991; Weitzner & McMillan, 1999). Although the majority of family caregivers adjust well, up to 30% of family caregivers, particularly those caring for patients with advanced disease, will have significant psychological distress (Weitzner *et al.*, 1999).

Patients require varying degrees of assistance. Assistance might be needed in activities of daily living, emotional needs, insurance or financial needs, transport, meal preparation or housekeeping. These needs for assistance can become overwhelming and increasingly complex and can cause an increase of caregiver burden. The distress of the family might also increase because more and more care is provided in the outpatient clinic and at home. From the literature it is known that the more time the caregiver spends on needs of the patient, the more the caregiver's schedule is altered and the more the caregiver experiences emotional distress (Stetz & Hanson, 1992; Yang & Kirscling, 1992; Give & Stommel, 1993). As a result, support for the family caregivers with adequate attention to their quality of life should be regarded as important aspects of palliative care. Although research has documented the burden and distress of family caregivers, little work has evaluated the impact of care giving on quality of life.

Weitzner *et al.* (1999) compared the impact of cancer care giving in curative and palliative care settings on family caregiver quality of life. Family caregivers of patients receiving palliative care had significantly lower QOL scores and lower scores on physical health than caregivers from the curative setting. The results from the study suggest that the lower QOL scores of caregivers in the palliative setting are a reflection of the patients' poorer performance status. The lower physical health scores of caregivers in the palliative setting appear to be a reflection of their lower educational level.

Only a few valid and reliable scales, specific for palliative care, were found to measure quality of life of the family. A promising example is the caregiver quality of life index – cancer. This measure consists of 35 items using a 5-point Likert-type scale to assess QOL in the family caregiver of cancer patients. The psychometric properties of this measure are promising. Test/retest reliability was 0.95 and internal consistency was 0.91 (Weitzner & McMillan, 1999). The instrument also has good convergent validity with other QOL and emotional distress measures and divergent validity with measures of physical health, social support and social desirability. The instrument seems also to be responsive to changes.

Ferrell (in Doyle *et al.*, 1998) developed a questionnaire for family caregivers analogue to a questionnaire used to assess patients' quality of life. It includes 27 items in four dimensions (physical well being, psychological well being, social concerns and spiritual well being). A numeric rating scale 0–10 is used. No information was found about the psychometric properties of this scale.

Since family quality of life is an important issue in palliative care, additional research is needed to examine the effect of specific care giving demands on caregiver quality of life through the palliative care trajectory and after the death of the family member. Studies should also focus on demographic, relational and psychological factors, which might determine caregivers' quality of life. This might be helpful in order to detect vulnerable or risk groups and to develop (preventive) intervention programmes for caregivers. More research into the validity and reliability of measurement instruments on caregiver quality of life is warranted.

9.6 Conclusions

Measuring quality of life and outcomes of the care of patients is important for several reasons. Clinical monitoring is important and needs detailed information about the patient in order to improve and aid patient care. Another purpose is to audit the care and determine whether standards of care are being achieved. Outcome measures can also be used to compare services and interventions or to assess the efficacy or cost-effectiveness of services. The measures described in this chapter fulfil these objectives in varying degrees. None of them meet all the objectives and it is questionable whether any tool could or should.

As yet there is no golden standard for assessing quality of life in palliative care. There is a need to continue research and development of valid and reliable instruments which include the most important dimensions of quality of life in terminally ill patients and their families and which are easy to use, in both inpatient and outpatient settings. Special attention should be paid to methodological and practical problems in measurement in this vulnerable group of patients. Since in palliative care the unit of care is patient and family, more attention should be paid to measures that focus on the quality of life of relatives.

Measurement instruments that itemise problems or issues of quality of life can provide a systematic way to ensure that patients' needs or distress and all domains of palliative care are addressed. Instruments cannot take the place of clinical interviews but they can focus and expedite them (Brady & Cella, 1999). By means of these instruments it is also possible to prioritise clinical care based on patients' own assessments. Structured assessments can also provide a way of communicating with patients and their families about difficult topics. Monitoring symptoms and problems might be helpful in assessing whether or not outcomes are achieved and to observe changes within or between patients.

Chapter 10

Evaluation of Palliative Care Services: Problems, Pitfalls and Recommendations

Huda Huijer Abu-Saad

10.1   Introduction

Palliative care services aim to meet the physical, emotional, social and spiritual needs of people who are terminally ill. These aims create a challenging task for evaluation studies in this area. Naturally, the concept of a good death becomes of great value. The question which then arises is whether people receiving specialised palliative care services have a better death. Indeed, what is meant by a good death, who judges a good death, and how can one actually know whether it did happen? A good death can be visualised in different ways depending on the source of information used. Health professionals may hold a different view of what death should be like from that held by the patients themselves. The task of evaluation could thus be seen as focusing on the processes of care that lead up to death and how these are interpreted by the different parties involved in the care process, mainly the patient, the immediate family and the health professional.

The difficulties facing the researcher of palliative care are numerous, but they can be divided into those which relate to the methodology used and the ethics of conducting research in this area, and those involving the extent to which outcome measures used and results achieved could be useful for evaluation purposes.

10.2   Methodology issues

In designing evaluation studies of palliative care services, investigators have to deal in general with a number of issues. Attrition due to early death, problems with recruitment and a low compliance rate for completion of questionnaires were cited by McWhinney *et al.* (1994) as reasons for not attaining the required sample size for adequate statistical power in their randomised controlled trial using a waiting list control group. In addition, opposition to randomisation by patients and referral sources, ethical problems raised by randomisation of dying patients, and the difficulties of collecting data from sick or exhausted patients may contribute to some of the difficulties in conducting trials. One of the main ethical problems is the denial of a service or treatment to the control group. It is also difficult to avoid exposure of the control group to the experimental effect. Moreover, dilution of the experimental effect may occur if patients randomised to hospice care were cared for on general wards when hospice beds were full (Kane *et al.*, 1984). Contamination and confounding, commonly encountered in palliative care research, could provide major threats to the validity of studies in this area. Factors related to diagnosis and personality as well as the perception of pain and other symptoms and ways of coping could confound the study results. Furthermore, the outcomes chosen for assessment may not be sensitive enough to capture the benefits of the service, and the timing of the different measurements may lead to under-recording of the effects of the intervention. Finally, the difficulty patients and caregivers may encounter in completing questionnaires may present another problem that the researcher has to deal with in conducting such studies.

Randomised controlled trials are not only impractical for palliative care services, they are also time-consuming and emotionally stressful for service providers. Perhaps this is why so few of them have been conducted. Non-randomised controlled trials using matched controls, with data collected by interviews with patients and care providers, are more common. They do, however, have a number of flaws: patients selecting hospice care may be fundamentally different from those choosing conventional care; and the suitability of controls is to a great extent a matter of judgement. Studies using comparisons before and after introducing palliative care are also subject to bias from secular changes in the health care system. Nevertheless, these designs do avoid the problem of the recruitment of patients, and problems regarding differences between groups can be controlled statistically. Before and after studies can be enhanced by including a thorough description of the developments and changes occurring during the project.

Rinck *et al.* (1997) identified a number of methodological issues in their systematic review of effectiveness research on palliative care. The review included 11 randomised clinical trials on comprehensive palliative care. Problems included the recruitment of study population in ten trials; its homogeneity in six; patient attrition in four; defining and maintaining the contrasts in interventions in six; and selection of outcome variables in four. In two studies, the problems were severe enough that no results could be reported. The authors conclude by stressing the importance of precise documentation of the process of care, the appropriate choice of outcome measures, and linking patient outcomes to the quality of care.

To evaluate the effectiveness of individual therapies in palliative care, randomised controlled trials are the best method to use. The number of patients eligible for entry into a particular trial is, however, very small. Multi-centre trials and n-of-1 trials have been suggested as ways of retaining the experimental method while overcoming the problem of patient recruitment. Multi-centre trials are important in evaluating drug therapies. The n-of-1 trial on the other hand is more suitable when the patient condition is relatively stable and with patients who are not imminently terminally ill. Exploration of this methodology is recommended in palliative care research; the n-of-1 trials may prove to be a robust method for evaluation research in this area. In addition to circumventing the problems of recruitment, they will provide the clinicians with scientifically sound evidence and confidence in their management decisions (Guyatt *et al.*, 1990).

Of paramount importance in palliative care research is the development and testing of specific outcome measures. The majority of the tools that are currently in use have been developed for other patient populations and only a small number has been tested in terminally ill patients. It is therefore recommended that available instruments be further tested for their validity, reliability and clinical utility in palliative care. It is highly likely that terminally ill patients could be overburdened by filling in long questionnaires. As a consequence and in order to spare the patient from further unnecessary burden, family members could be used as proxies. Caution should, however, be exercised when using proxies; their assessments could differ from those of patients. The concordance between patients, home carers and professional carers is an area of research that is becoming increasingly important in palliative care and so warrants future attention.

10.3   Qualitative methods

The emphasis placed on measurable outcomes in palliative care research and on the quantitative representation of patients' perceptions of their condition and of the care given can be frustrating to the researcher, the patient and the caregivers. This emphasis contradicts the goals of palliative care which are in general patient-centred, tailored to the needs of the patient and family, and multidimensional and interdisciplinary. This approach acknowledges the uniqueness of each patient and serves as a quality indicator of palliative care services. This variability in meeting the unique needs of patients is, on the other hand, a major source of confounding in experimental studies.

As an alternative to the rigid approach using questionnaires, patient concerns may be elicited through qualitative methods such as interviews, relatively structured or fairly unstructured, as well as participant observations of the care provided to the patient. These qualitative research methods provide more in-depth information on the meaning and perception of illness, satisfaction and preference, and processes of care. Exploring the beliefs that terminally ill patients have about their illness is an important area of research in palliative care. Through this approach one may unravel the beliefs patients have about life and death, related symptom tolerance and expectations of care. A number of authors have used this methodology to explore patients' meaning of pain (Ferrel *et al.*, 1993) and quality of life (Bertero & Ek, 1993) in advanced stage cancer. Results obtained point to the diversity of the patients' experiences and needs in both areas. Uncovering the meaning of pain and quality of life that patients hold can lead to ways in which each patient may best be helped and thus to the identification of tailor-made interventions.

Patient satisfaction with palliative care services is a difficult and rather controversial area of research. It is nevertheless a central concept in evaluation research. Field's (1994) review of patient satisfaction with terminal care provides a comprehensive summary of the methodological and practical difficulties of this kind of research in general. Qualitative research methods have been used to assess patient satisfaction with information given with regard to diagnosis, prognosis and treatment options. Interestingly, although emphasis in palliative care is placed on the importance of open communication, the way communication is managed may vary from culture to culture. Centeno-Cortes & Nunez-Olante (1994) found that only 32% of the patients with advanced malignant cancer in Spain had been informed of their diagnosis. This contrasts with a study conducted by Coughlan (1993) in Ireland who found most patients to be informed of their diagnosis.

The structured observation of care encounters is another method used in evaluating palliative care encounters and interactions between patients, family and health professionals. Many of the studies have focused on the staff perspectives of the care process. Raudonis (1993) took the patient's perspective into consideration when studying the empathetic relationship between nurse and patient. Empathetic relationships were described by patients to include 'acknowledging the patient's personhood', 'approaching the patients as people with an illness rather than as ill people', and 'reciprocating by sharing feelings and experiences'. Observational studies can provide extensive descriptions of complex social relationships, and describe the atmosphere of a particular institution. Hence, they can reveal and highlight examples of good practice and point out areas of concern where improvement is needed (Robbins, 1998).

Another method in evaluating palliative care is the responsive and reflexive approach to evaluation. The underlying assumption of this method is the focus on narratives, or 'telling the tale', that are used by people to interpret their past, present and anticipated experiences. According to Abma (2000), people commonly tell stories in order to understand what is happening to them. Different narratives are as a result produced *qua* form and content about a programme or service. The dynamics of the process of what people tell, the structure given to narrating these experiences and the ways ideas are communicated, are all relevant and important in responsive evaluation. Using interviews and participative observations one can gain an understanding of different points of view on the current practice of palliative care and the role of the different players in it (Abma, 2000). This method, although time-consuming and not free from criticism, does stimulate further reflection on palliative care research and offers insight into ways that can be used to enhance and improve palliative care services.

10.4   Prognosis issues

In addition to the above-mentioned difficulties regarding design, the questions regarding prognosis and comparative end-points are also essential in palliative care research. In this area of research, difficulty exists in defining when palliative care starts and when curative care ends. Despite the ambiguities encountered in defining the boundaries of palliative care, two methods have been used for assessing prognosis, mainly clinical judgement and prognostic indicators (Robbins, 1998). Both methods have their own limitations and are thus inconclusive in predicting prognosis and life expectancy. Maltoni *et al.* (1994) suggested a way forward via the development of a multidimensional prognostic index linked to biological and nutritional factors and performance status and symptoms. Such an index can not only be used for research purposes but can facilitate the planning of treatment and care packages in palliative care settings.

In 1999, Pirovano and others published the construction of a palliative prognostic score based on factors identified in a prospective multicentre study of 519 patients with a median survival of 32 days. The palliative prognostic score includes the following variables: clinical prediction of survival, Karnofsky performance status, anorexia, dyspnoea, total white blood count and lymphocyte percentage. Maltoni *et al.* (1995) validated this prognostic score for terminally ill cancer patients in order to determine its value in clinical practice. The palliative prognostic score was tested on 451 evaluable patients entered in the hospice programmes of 14 Italian palliative care centres. It was found to be able to subdivide the validation-independent case series into three risk groups. Median survival was 76 days in group A, 32 days in group B and 14 days in group C. The authors concluded that the palliative prognostic score is a simple instrument which permits a more accurate quantification of expected survival.

10.5   Ethical considerations

Few would question the need for conducting more research in this area, as long as it is appropriate and well designed. All clinical research needs to be conducted in an ethical manner, and with regard to palliative care research these issues operate with even more force because of the physical, emotional and cognitive frailty of the research participants. Since the majority of palliative care services are provided to people with cancer, the complex fears and anxieties that accompany the cancer diagnosis should be taken into consideration when entering this sensitive area of research. A large number of people do not like to reflect on their experiences with cancer, they do not like to admit to the seriousness of their disease, and in some cases they would like to stay in denial of the imminent approach of death. The question of whether it is ethical to carry out such studies in these situations needs to be raised regularly and the benefits to be achieved need to be weighed carefully.

10.6   Conclusions and recommendations

In summary, no single method can be fully free from flaws. Investigators are encouraged to use different methods or a combination of methods in designing palliative care studies. The chosen method will depend on the question being raised and the audience being addressed.

The necessity of developing palliative care research programmes has been recognised for a number of years. This is particularly related to the expansion of services in this area and to the priorities set by policy makers in the health care sector for efficient and effective evidence-based care. As a result, evaluation of the services provided will no longer be considered a luxury but a must.

Based on the analysis provided in the preceding chapters with regard to palliative care services for adults and children, a number of recommendations have been formulated where research is still warranted. All the recommendations are equally applicable to adult and paediatric palliative care research:

- Studies addressing effectiveness and efficacy are best addressed using quantitative research designs. Multi-centre trials and n-of-1 trials are recommended as ways of retaining the experimental method while overcoming the problem of patient recruitment.
- Instruments used in effectiveness studies need to be psychometrically tested for use in palliative care.
- Studies aimed at identifying patients' problems and needs as well as satisfaction with care and with services provided are better tackled using qualitative methodologies.
- Researchers interested in the experiences of patients, family members and health professionals are better off using qualitative designs.
- Of particular importance in evaluation research is the linking of process variables with patient outcomes. This particular area of research has not been adequately researched and deserves to be addressed in the future.
- In addition to a controlled study, an audit of charts as well as a survey of users can be conducted. For policy purposes and in order to make decisions about a single service, it is recommended to study palliative care using different designs and on the basis of different perspectives.
- Evaluation of palliative care services for children is practically non-existent and as a result warrants future attention.
- Of interest is the impact of palliative care services on symptom management. A state-of-the-art study addressing the magnitude of this impact in palliative care is recommended.
- Quality of life constitutes a major area of emphasis in palliative care and deserves more attention in future research.
- The meaning of death, how patients and family members cope with it, and the support they need in the process are areas warranting future research as well.
- Studies evaluating support services to meet the needs of health care professionals in palliative care deserve more attention in future research.

Chapter 11

Bridging the Evidence to Clinical Practice: A Glimpse at Future Challenges in Palliative Care

Huda Huijer Abu-Saad

11.1 Introduction

This chapter is intended to bring more insight into the state of the art with regard to developments in palliative care in general. It provides the reader with more factual information on what we know based on evidence and how the knowledge can be bridged to the clinical setting. It is meant to set the stage as well for future developments in this growing field of care. In order to accomplish this task, the chapter will first begin with some reflections on the principles and practices of palliative care. Secondly, emphasis will be placed on summarising the evidence presented in this book on aspects such as transitions in palliative care, effectiveness and efficacy of different models of care, needs assessment, pain and symptom management, and tools to evaluate palliative care service provisions. Thirdly, some reflections will be made with regard to service provision and policy issues. Finally, this chapter will give a glimpse into the future challenges facing palliative care.

11.2 Reflections on palliative care

As we have seen in the introduction and the succeeding chapters of this book, the term 'palliative' historically refers to the words 'shield' and 'cloak'. Morris (1997) argues that the term with its pejorative connotations was associated with quackery, cloaking, covering up and disguising of symptoms, while the disease is left untouched. On the other hand, and set against these pejorative and negative associations, palliative was also described to mean 'skin' or 'hide'. These terms have more of a positive connotation and symbolise an active role and a heroic act on the part of the caregiver to protect and shield the patient from unnecessary harm.

Paradigmatic views

The notion of palliative care, based on the above discussions, continues to be associated with the concealment and relief of symptoms suffered by people who cannot be cured (Doyle, 1994). This perspective presents paradigmatic views that typify current medical care and health care practices. Disease, according to this view, is seen as a series of symptoms that need to be addressed in a paternalistic, linear and problem-solving fashion in order to cure the patient. Palliative care is on the other hand broader and more holistic. According to many, palliative care needs as a result to differentiate itself from mainstream health care practices by focusing on the notions and premises of the concept 'care'.

The concept of 'care' on the other hand has been associated with a multitude of meanings and nuances and may mean different things to different people. Of particular interest in palliative care is the description of the concept 'care' provided by Clark and Seymour (1999). According to the authors, care directs attention from paternalism by focusing more on participation of the person and family in the care process. Furthermore, care puts more emphasis on holism and less on linearity in assessing and managing the health care concerns and problems of patients and their home carers. Finally, care focuses on the person in their totality and not alone on the patient who happens to be terminally ill. Caring for a person in the terminal phase of illness denotes compassion for the whole person and family as well as a total integration of the care process, which remains to a large extent fragmented in our health care delivery system.

The above descriptions, and in particular the associations of palliative care with care and caring, are not meant to exclude and monopolise 'caring' as a distinct characteristic of palliative care. As Ahmedzai (1993b) rightfully suggests, caring and curing are not mutually exclusive activities; each is an integral part of the other. The roles of medicine and nursing in this activity should be regarded as complementary rather than competitive and demarcated. Emphasis is placed in this model on interdisciplinary teamwork, on breaking the barriers between disciplines, and most importantly on achieving a balance between caring and curing activities.

Good death

Closely related to the principles and practices of palliative care is the notion of a 'good death'. Some historians argue that impersonalisation, technological advancements and the domination of death by professionals have become particular features of modern death. The counterparts to this development have focused on the issues prevailing in a 'good death', which involve the notions of 'open awareness', 'truth telling', 'expression of feelings', and having a 'sense of meaning and trust'. These issues become of paramount importance when new subjectivity within the health care system prevails, where patients are assessed not only on the basis of their disease and the ensuing physical symptoms and needs, but also in relation to their personal, psychosocial and spiritual concerns.

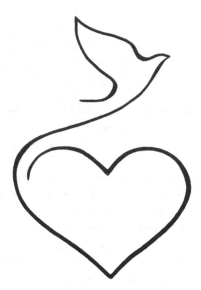

Fig. 11.1   Symbol of palliative care (Courtesy of Simon Andras, Budapest)

A 'good death' according to Kellehear (1990) means 'beautiful death, the ideal and the exemplary'. Death continues to be an important feature of cultural life surrounded by all its mystical aspects, prescribed behaviours and expected modes of transcendental being. Field *et al.* (1997) studied the ways death is experienced and expressed among men and women of different cultures. A central theme emerged in their analysis emphasising the crucial role of the social context and the wider cultural environment in shaping the meaning of death and dying to the individual. Death is seen as a private and individual encounter, which takes place within the boundaries of one's own home, family and culture. Rituals associated with death and dying are religious, prescriptive and publicly acknowledged. They emphasise in many ways the stability of one's world and the certainty of the life-death trajectory. Control over nature and the will to change life's natural pattern is seen as impossible and unnecessary. The romantic notions of the beauty of a peaceful death play a major role in this respect. This picture is contrasted with hospitalised death, which is characterised by a loss of individual choice, fear, isolation from family and friends, and by being totally impersonal.

The developments in palliative care and in particular the hospice movement have contributed to a large extent towards changing our views on what a good death is and should be. They have promoted in other words the ideologies of the good death, which were lost to many in the process of medicalisation of the end of life and ultimately the impersonalisation of death itself. The developments in palliative care, although of great value, were not always obtainable when it came to achieving the goal of a 'good death'. For many, death continues to be seen as far from 'good' or 'good enough' and as such unwanted and feared. These issues will continue to create a challenge for palliative care services and one needs as a result to confront them with diligence, wisdom and balance.

The ethics of dying

It is difficult to address the issues of palliative care without making reference to the large number of current articles, writings and commentaries on euthanasia. For many countries in the world, and more specifically the USA, Australia and the Netherlands, these have become major issues for public and political debate and in some cases have led to the institution of policy in this area. The debates have their roots in the public's doubt and mistrust with regard to the limits of medicine and technology in prolonging life and in extending the life expectancy beyond one's own will. They also stem from the public's fear that professionals could have the utmost power in controlling and influencing end-of-life decision-making. The debates in this area can only be seen as a reflection of the many uncertainties with which our modern society is struggling regarding end-of-life, and death and dying issues.

The debates over euthanasia rage at the moment with rhetoric, for example concerning 'self-determination', 'choice', and in 'the patient's best interest'. These discussions could mask in some cases the prevailing anxiety about medical rationing being applied covertly to some marginal groups of our society such as the elderly, the disabled and the cognitively impaired (Clark & Seymour, 1999). As the debates rage in many countries of the world, multitudes of definitions have come into existence reflecting the tensions and disagreements around this significant social issue. Terms such as voluntary (active) euthanasia, involuntary (passive) euthanasia, slow euthanasia, physician-assisted suicide, withdrawal of treatment, and advanced directive (living will) are among the many used as synonyms of euthanasia.

The current debate over euthanasia, according to Howarth and Jefferys (1996), has to do, at least partly, with the 'agency' issue. In other words, it is concerned with who does and who should control the decisions to hasten or procure death. Of particular importance in this respect are the roles of the individual and society, and the interface between the two, that determine how euthanasia is seen and practised. This will eventually have an influence and impact on the thinking with regard to effective symptom management and palliative care. Within such a context, it is highly unlikely that a consensus will be reached with respect to end-of-life ethics. The ethical debates will surely continue and it is projected that the mosaic of euthanasia issues will as a result flourish. Of particular importance to palliative care is that the public is adequately informed over the multitude of facets that can impinge on ethical issues and decisions in this area.

11.3   The research evidence

The research evidence summarised in this book provides the fundamental cornerstones for the discussions and conclusions presented in this section. In addition, a number of clinical practice guidelines have been consulted and where appropriate have been referenced. Due to the complexity of the subject matter presented and in some cases the lack of strong evidence, no grading will be given to the selections made. However, and in order to do justice to the content under discussion, recommendations for practice will be made based on the presented evidence. The strength of the recommendations made can be found in the different chapters of this book.

In order for us to discuss the research evidence comprehensively, it is imperative that the aims and principles of palliative care are briefly listed. In addition to the aims and principles of palliative care cited in a number of chapters of this book, a number of statements listed by the Working Party on Clinical Guidelines in Palliative Care (1997) have been either added to or in some cases integrated into the text.

The aims of palliative care can be summarised, as a result, as follows:

- To consider the patient and family as the centre of care
- To help relieve as promptly and effectively as possible the most prevailing symptoms
- To ensure that the quality of remaining life of the patient is not adversely affected
- To provide support and encouragement to the home carers and informal carers of the patient
- To support the professional carers in providing effective patient-tailored care
- To enable and make it possible for the patients in palliative care to die in the place of their choosing, if at all feasible
- To support the family and the bereaved parents and siblings with bereavement issues
- To minimise the morbidity associated with bereavement.

The principles of palliative care can be stated as follows:

- Emphasis is placed on patient and family participation in the care process. Patient- and family-centered palliative care is the motto of care and applies as much to adults as to children.
- A collaborative and multiprofessional approach by health care professionals in palliative care constitutes the norm rather than the exception.
- Effective symptom management is of paramount importance. Medication use should be adequate, developmentally appropriate, individually tailored and regularly administered to relieve and prevent prevailing symptoms.
- Ongoing assessment and regular monitoring of support services provided to the family as a unit, are available on a 24-hour basis. Possibilities for back-up emergency services, in case of need, are available.
- Access and early referral to specialist palliative care services are available for both patients and their families, if needed.

Prognostic issues in palliative care

Currently there are no clear-cut guidelines demarcating when curative care stops and palliative care begins. The decisions made in this area are mostly based on personal and professional experience and less on empirical evidence. Progress in the field, however, remains promising. A number of prognostic indexes have been developed and are potentially of value. However, they are not adequately tested on their usability and acceptability by the clinicians and on their clinical relevance for the practice setting. This issue remains of crucial importance in palliative care practice and research.

Transitional issues in palliative care

This is closely related to the prognostic issues mentioned earlier. Many health professionals struggle with these issues on a daily basis in their clinical practice. When should one stop treatment and begin palliation? Is there such a demarcating line between the two? Should palliative care begin at the moment of diagnosis or only when cure is no longer possible? How much can palliative care go hand in hand with curative care? Can the patient receive curative treatments when already in palliative care? How invasive can these treatments be? These questions can go on and on.

Transitional models in palliative care do, however, exist for both children and adults. Their value for the practice setting has been shown time after time. We would strongly recommend as a result that these models be used when managing the life-threatening illnesses of both children and adults. They can prove to be of help to the clinicians as well as the family when treatment and prognosis issues are mentioned and fully discussed.

Patient and family participation

The aims and principles of palliative care emphasise the involvement of the patient, adult and child, and the family in the care process. Collaborative decision-making with regard to treatment and provision of other required services is made in close consultation with the patient and family. There is evidence, however, based on comparative studies and use of proxies, that family members and home carers do not always tell the same story as the patients themselves. They are less capable, for instance, of assessing the patients' symptoms accurately and in particular those of anxiety and depression, and are inclined to be more negative about quality of life issues and in particular the quality of the care provided. Nevertheless, information obtained from family members about the experience of terminal illness can be very valuable, especially in those cases where getting patients' accounts of the situation is practically impossible. In particular, home carers can provide important information on the adequacy of pain management and symptom control, and on the prompt and diligent responses of the health and social services directly involved in the care of the patient. Both patients and family carers have important stories to tell when it comes to palliative care issues. It is as a result important to listen to both stories if a fuller picture of the care process needs to be made.

Assessment of patients' needs

There is evidence suggesting that the perception of family members or home carers and professional carers varies from that of patients, especially with regard to the severity and management of symptoms. Patients' accounts of their own situation are as a result recommended. Health professionals need to remember that patients who do not report the presence of a symptom spontaneously are not necessarily symptom-free. Inquiry should be made in particular about less obvious symptoms such as nausea, constipation and fatigue. Many distresses can be inferred from non-verbal cues and health professionals need to be aware of clues such as grimacing when touched or moved, or the agitation associated with tachypnoea.

The assessment of the psychological state of the patient can be of tremendous value. Evidence suggests that patients have heightened fears and anxieties about the escalation of some symptoms. For example, the increase in pain severity may be seen by the patient to lead to breathing problems and to the cessation of breathing in particular during sleep, and they may feel that the administration of morphine may hasten death. Evidence suggests as well that anxiety is common in terminal illness. It is related to the patient's lack of knowledge about the diagnosis and eventual prognosis. Anxiety is commonly associated with certain symptoms such as dyspnoea, dysphagia and sudden haemorrhage. Adequate support and accurate information about the disease trajectory and the anticipated symptoms may allay some of these fears and anxieties.

In addition to the above, an assessment of the patient's expectations and views on what a 'good death' means, of their religious and cultural beliefs, of their spirituality and value systems is seen as essential if patient-centered holistic and participative quality palliative care is to be provided.

Systematic assessment tools such as the McGill questionnaire and the Support Team Assessment Schedule (STAS) can be helpful in obtaining a comprehensive assessment. Care should be taken, however, not to overburden the patient with lengthy tools which can sometimes be irrelevant if the patient's illness is at its latest stage. There is evidence from observational studies that the above mentioned symptoms and problems are often encountered by patients in the terminal phase of their illness. The process of assessment, however, has not been adequately looked at in comparative studies. As a result more research is warranted in this area.

Assessment of family members' needs

In the provision of care, the involvement of the family, as discussed earlier, is of paramount importance. The burden of care on the family, however, should not be underestimated. When dealing with terminally ill children, the situation can become more extreme. There is evidence suggesting that parents can feel isolated, lonely, depressed and bewildered by the experience. Adequate support, the availability of a back-up system in case of an emergency and the provision of respite care are seen as important, especially when palliative care is provided at home.

There is also evidence suggesting that caring for a terminally ill patient at home may have detrimental effects on the family carers' lives. The psychological, emotional, social and financial burdens are quite high. Fatigue, anxiety and depression and concerns over the family structure, its continuity and integrity, as well as financial concerns, are commonly reported. Regular assessment and ongoing monitoring of the needs and concerns of these families are as a result essential.

Assessment of professional carers' needs

An important aspect in palliative care is the assessment of the professional carers' needs. This area has not been adequately addressed in palliative care. There is some evidence suggesting that working with dying patients and having to cope with death and dying on a day-to-day basis can be emotionally burdening for professional carers. Stress and burnout among staff working in hospice and other palliative care settings have been found to be high. Staff support and stress-intervention methods have received as a result considerable attention in palliative care.

Apart from formal staff support, aspects of teamwork and working in specialist palliative care teams have been found to be related to higher job satisfaction and to lower levels of stress. There is evidence suggesting that levels of stress can be lowered through the provision of appropriate levels of education and adequate skill training. The acquisition of new knowledge in general is known to increase feelings of confidence in one's work, an aspect intimately connected to feelings of stress and anxiety. In-service training and professional development courses are as a result fundamental to building staff confidence, lowering stress and burnout levels, and ultimately improving the quality of care provided.

Pain and symptom management

The primary aim of symptom management in palliative care is to control the symptoms, which are distressing to the patient, tailoring all therapy to the patient's needs. A treatment plan for the management of symptoms in children and adults needs to be developed and put to use. Such a plan needs to be based on the most recent evidence for the management of a specific symptom. Clinical practice guidelines developed by expert working parties and by the WHO need to be used (WHO 1990, 1998; Working Party on Clinical Guidelines in Palliative Care 1997, 1998). They should define what should be given, how often, using which route, and what should be done in case of breakthrough of a symptom. The oral route is preferable if the patient has no difficulty swallowing and there is no danger of aspiration. When this time comes, however, the subcutaneous route should be used instead. Injections should not be given intramuscularly either to children or adults, especially those who are cachectic. The rectal route is an alternative but is rather less convenient or acceptable to most patients. The parenteral route can be used as a last resort when all other possibilities have been exhausted.

The management of pain should be tailored for each patient. The treatment should be based on a logical approach, starting at the level most appropriate to the patient's level of pain and progressing to the next step if the pain cannot be controlled. The WHO three-step analgesic ladder is of particular use for the management of pain in children and adults. Analgesics need to be prescribed and administered on a regular basis to control pain, prevent its exacerbation and prevent it from recurring. Regular monitoring of the treatment needs to be carried out through regular contacts with patient and family, including: assessing the efficacy of medications, monitoring for side effects, detecting new pains and assessing related psychosocial problems. The use of a pain diary has been found to be helpful for patients and family. Regular recording of information in a pain diary may be helpful to the clinicians as well in monitoring the progression of pain and the effectiveness of the treatment plan. There is adequate evidence supporting the effectiveness of the WHO three-step analgesic ladder in managing pain, in particular in adults. Some evidence based on anecdotal case studies and observational studies is available as well in children.

Of particular interest is the use of non-pharmacological therapies in conjunction with pharmacological therapies in the management of pain and other symptoms. Some evidence is found attesting to their effectiveness in palliative care. There is some evidence that patients may benefit from physical measures such as transcutaneous nerve stimulation and acupuncture. Psychosocial interventions such as the use of imagery, relaxation, distraction and hypnosis have been found to be helpful in relieving procedural pain and anxiety. Obviously, more work needs to be conducted in this important field of study.

Models of care

In Chapter 5 a comprehensive description is given of a total of 48 studies conducted in the field of palliative care. Few of these studies are population-based and give prevalence figures on the preference and actual place of death in different countries. The majority address effectiveness and efficacy issues related to the different palliative care services provided. Some studies have compared terminal care in a variety of settings such as acute care hospitals, home, hospice, specialist palliative care units, specialist palliative care teams and long-term residential and nursing home institutions.

Evidence has shown that pain and symptom control and family support were found to be more effective in hospices and specialised palliative care units. Most terminally ill patients who can express a choice initially want to die at home. Terminal care is possible and preferable at home. Palliative care provided at home was found to be more cost-effective when compared to hospital care. There is evidence suggesting that carers at home need more information about available services and help lines. They also need support from health professionals in dealing with the day-to-day issues of terminal illness. Evidence also suggests that health professionals need to be aware and have a better appreciation of the problems encountered by patients and families at home. In a number of studies it was shown that patients receiving specialised palliative care at home are able to spend more time with their families at home and eventually do die at home.

In general, when palliative care services were compared with conventional care, improvements were found in pain and symptom management and in quality of life. In addition, there was an increase in patient and family satisfaction with care, and a reduction in costs was found. There is evidence to suggest that conventional care alone is inadequate in meeting the needs of terminally ill patients and their families. The review also points out that a multiprofessional palliative care team can be very effective in meeting the needs of patients and their families and in providing access to other services at home. There was evidence of increased satisfaction of patients and carers, better symptom control, reduction in hospital days, reduction in costs, more time spent at home by patients and increased likelihood of patients dying where they wished. The use of a multiprofessional palliative care team is found to have an impact on the quality of care delivered and on reducing the overall costs. More importantly, there is strong evidence to suggest that the co-ordination of services for terminally ill patients results in substantial cost savings.

Tools for evaluating palliative care

We have seen in the preceding sections the importance of being able to measure the effectiveness of palliative care and in particular the effectiveness of management plans in relieving pain and other ensuing symptoms. In order to do that effectively, one needs valid, reliable and clinically relevant assessment and measurement tools developed for this area. For evaluating the quality of palliative care, issues related to quality of life, functional ability, symptom management and patient satisfaction become important. A number of instruments have been found which were developed particularly for palliative care research. More information on these instruments is provided in Chapter 9. More work needs to be done, however, in developing, adapting and testing instruments to measure and assess pain and other symptoms. Questions related to tools developed to assess patient satisfaction with palliative care also need further attention in the future. One is led to believe that patients in palliative care require a different assessment approach. A tool needs to be not only valid, reliable and clinically relevant, but also simple, easy to use and requiring as little time as possible.

11.4   Reflections on service delivery and policy issues

In the previous section, the research evidence with regard to palliative care services is summarised and, depending on the state of the art of the evidence, recommendations are made for the practice setting. In this section, emphasis will be placed on implementation and policy issues with regard to service development and delivery now and in the future.

It is obvious that palliative care services increasingly flourished in the last two decades of the twentieth century. A large number of models and care services are being developed and introduced in the practice setting. All these models of care have the presumed goal of better meeting the needs of the terminally ill patients and their families. The expansion and diversification of palliative care into a wide variety of settings, such as the hospice, home, hospital, residential homes for the elderly and nursing homes, can be seen in many countries throughout the world. This diversification of services has created tensions between policy makers on the one hand and service providers on the other. The evolving relationship between the main actors in this sector is also influenced by the national agenda on health and social policy issues which determines to a large extent how palliative care services should be organised and delivered.

One should not forget during this proliferate period of growth that it was the charismatic enthusiasm and unrelenting efforts and dedication of a number of pioneers in palliative care that have brought the hospice movement to its present status. These pioneers managed to put terminal care and palliative care on the national agenda, to secure funding to establish hospices, and to bring about speciality areas in palliative medicine and palliative care. Their work was seen as pioneers' work then and as a challenge, mainly because they dared to oppose the normal stream of policy development in health care. In the UK for example, funding has been secured by charitable giving and the establishment of many hospices going hand in hand. Local groups were able to raise sufficient funds to build a hospice, which would be established as a visible sign of care within the community. This was seen as the highest level of giving by many. This led eventually to the rapid expansion of this sector, which was carried out in an unplanned way under the auspices of local authorities with less interference from health authorities at the national level. Such a development has led undoubtedly to tensions, which can only be resolved if and when a partnership based on a co-existence can be established between all parties involved.

Hospital-based palliative care also witnessed a very rapid growth in the same two decades, which has created in the process a major challenge for this sector. The hospital services, however, have varied considerably over the years. They vary in the extent to which they have multidisciplinary involvement, in the support they receive from health authorities, and in the established evidence of their efficacy. In a report by Seale and Kelly (1997), detailed analysis of comparative data was given on patients dying in a hospice or a nearby hospital. Results showed that in terms of symptom management hospital care was comparable to hospice care. Hospitals were found, however, to lag behind when it came to psychosocial care and communication skills. The hospital atmosphere is still seen as too rushed, very noisy and less patient- and family-centered.

On the other hand, palliative care at home, which is in a rapid state of expansion, has been widely supported by policy makers and health care providers in this field. It is also a stated health care policy goal of many governments throughout the world. This is by itself a worthwhile development and one that needs to be encouraged and nurtured. But despite all these efforts, we have seen a paradox developing in home palliative care. Although many people have a stated preference to die at home, very few actually achieve this goal. The lack of adequate support to the family and sometimes the lack of the special expertise expected of the health care professionals, have been regularly cited as reasons for this paradox. The multiplicity of available services also creates another dilemma. Palliative care provided at home can be offered by a wide variety of specialist and generic services such as primary health care teams, generic health care teams, specialist palliative care domiciliary services and hospice day care. The boundaries between the different services provided remains vague and to a large extent blurred. It is essential as a result that collaboration between health professionals in the different primary care settings and continued dialogue between service providers, takes place. This is regarded as an important cornerstone if home palliative care is to survive and continue to flourish.

Of particular significance in this discussion is the attention paid to residential homes for the elderly and to nursing homes as providers of palliative care services. Clearly both institutions have important roles to play in meeting the needs of a growing number of elderly people. However, major concerns continue to haunt this sector, which need to be resolved if quality palliative care is to be provided. These concerns have to do with the wide variability in the standards of care, in the quality of nursing and medical care, in the educational and skill level of staff, and in the ability of the staff to deal with death and dying issues. Furthermore, they have to do with issues related to work stress and availability of human resources. If residential and nursing homes are to play a role in palliative care, a number of conditions need to be met. First, they need to be included in the educational activities promoted by palliative care organisations. Second, they need to have better links with other providers of palliative care. Lastly, they need to put more emphasis on educational preparation and specialised training in recruiting and maintaining their staff. The current reliance on poorly paid and unskilled staff may be the fundamental barrier to the provision of quality palliative care services in both sectors.

Although we have seen a phenomenal growth in palliative care services over the last few decades, many of these developments can be seen as a piecemeal response to various local interests as well as to funding opportunities. This is in sharp contrast to initiatives being developed based on feasibility and needs assessment studies, which are ideally guided by national government-led policy rather than local policy. In some countries such as the Netherlands for instance, there is a commitment from the government to develop a national strategy, which is intended to guide the further development of palliative care at the national level. This is reflected in the establishment and funding of centres for palliative care throughout the country and in the co-ordination of the activities of these centres at the national level. Needs assessment studies using different methodologies could contribute immensely to shaping and guiding these developments and are as a result recommended.

However, and irrespective of how services are developed and delivered, the co-ordination of these services remains one of the most crucial aspects and one of paramount importance in palliative care. As terminally ill patients and their families move between the different settings and health care agencies, they need the support and guidance of a health care professional familiar with their situation, who can co-ordinate their care. It is envisioned, based on policy development in this field, that the primary caregiver, in this case either the family physician or the nurse, will be able to take on this role in the future.

11.5   Challenges facing palliative care in the future

This section will address a number of areas commonly seen as challenges for the field in the future. First, some general propositions about palliative care are presented. Second, specific challenges with regard to service provision, policy issues, public and professional education, ethical concerns and spiritual care are presented. Finally, recommendations are made on 'where do we go from here?' in the field of palliative care.

General propositions

Developments in palliative care have shown that the concept is not only fluid and versatile but also context and culture-bound. According to Clark and Seymour (1999), it is important to keep in mind that palliative care arises in the context of religious pluralism, scepticism over medicine, health care consumerism, and reflexivity in the body and the self. As such, palliative care has provided health care with a new ethos and has produced a new ethic of care for the dying. Despite these developments, one should not forget the challenges facing palliative care in keeping up with a rapidly developing field. Palliative care needs as a result to become reflexive, analysing its strengths and weaknesses and at the same time staying abreast of, while engaging in the discussions around, actual issues in this field. Palliative care needs, in other words, to take part and engage openly in the current philosophical and ethical debates around end-of-life issues and in particular euthanasia. These ongoing developments create a challenge for palliative care which necessitates continued reflections into its ideologies in relation to society and the population it serves.

In order for palliative care to develop and mature into a well-recognised speciality in health care, ambiguities with regard to definitions, purpose and mission need to be resolved. Discussions are ongoing worldwide with regard to the meanings of the different terms currently in use in palliative care. Doyle (1994) believes that palliative care, terminal care and hospice care are interchangeable terms, all meaning the same. On the other hand, the working party of the National Council for Hospice and Specialist Palliative Care Services, in its report on definitions, makes a distinction between the different terminologies used in palliative care (NCHSPCS, 1995). Terminal care is seen, for example, as part of palliative care, while the term hospice care is completely abandoned from the lexicon in the field. By far the greatest clarity is needed when it comes to the term palliative care and the elements that constitute its service provision. Public and professional education here remains of paramount importance. These issues are seen as major challenges for the field in the future.

Service provision

Of particular importance worldwide, and certainly a challenge in the field of palliative care, is the availability of human resources. The success of any palliative care service depends to a large extent on the availability of the needed physical, instrumental and human resources and to a large extent on the willingness of policy makers to fulfil these requirements. Palliative care provided by hospitals, hospices, nursing homes, and in the home setting should be seen as an integral part of health care services in all countries. The importance of developing the best methods to meet the needs of terminally ill children, adults and their families remains a challenge for professionals in this field. The type and appropriateness of services provided and the quality of methods used are in this respect considered crucial. A national policy on service provision and funding is critical. The challenge for palliative care in the future is to make this happen.

Public education

Public education is one of the areas in palliative care that has not received adequate attention. The general public is to a large extent unfamiliar with the term, let alone the purpose and mission of palliative care. This is an area of great concern. The importance of the lay public should not be underestimated, especially when it comes to campaigning for comprehensive and humane treatment on issues dealing with suffering and death and dying in children and adults. The public needs to be educated with regard to service provision and treatment modalities in palliative care. They need to be aware that pain and other symptoms can be effectively relieved and their loved ones need not suffer unnecessarily; that the use of opioid drugs is safe and effective in children and adults, when used appropriately for pain control; and that the appropriate use of opioid drugs does not lead to abuse and addiction and, when adequately administered, does not lead to shortening life. These issues create a challenge for palliative care that should not be taken lightly.

Professional education

Despite the proliferation of knowledge in palliative care and the research evidence currently available, serious challenges remain in clinical practice. The gap between knowledge and practice grows continually. Health care professionals in general lack up-to-date information and current evidence on effective means to manage pain and other symptoms in adults and children. These facts put the issue of professional education on the top priority list in palliative care. The highest priority now and in the future must be the application of existing knowledge to clinical practice. Emphasis should be placed on integrating evidence into the curricula of health care professionals such as medicine, nursing and psychology. The guidelines that are currently available through the WHO and other recognised professional bodies should be made available to all educational institutions both in developed and developing countries. In addition, similar information should be provided through continuing education and intensive training programmes for health care workers in the field. Professional certification should be available and should be required of all practitioners in the field of palliative care. Finally, emphasis should be placed on ways of changing practice through changing the organisational culture and the behaviour of the individual clinician. All of these aspects are without doubt difficult to achieve but nevertheless important in providing high-level quality care in this area of practice – a challenge that palliative care should continue addressing with a great deal of diligence.

Ethical issues

The true primary ethical principles in clinical practice are to do good (beneficence) and to minimise harm (nonmaleficence). This means that one needs to seek a balance between the benefits and burdens of treatment in children and adults alike. These principles are founded in respect for the person's own decisions with regard to how much treatment should be given and how much of the treatment can be tolerated. The infliction of excessive pain and suffering on children and adults should not be justified by the aggressiveness of the therapies to treat the disease and its sequel. The person's right to choose is here of particular importance. Health care professionals should be the patients' advocates in this respect. They should practice the humane and competent treatment of pain and suffering, particularly when it concerns a dying child. In many countries in the world, most financial resources are directed towards the aggressive treatment of disease, in other words the curative therapies. Very limited resources are available as a result for palliative therapies. Misuse of resources represents a problem worldwide, especially when these therapies do not necessarily lead to a cure or to improvement in the quality of the person's life. A large chunk of these resources could be redirected towards programmes which put emphasis on pain relief and palliative care. Collaborative efforts initiated by the WHO and professional organisations worldwide might help shift the balance. This is an area where palliative care can be challenged to look beyond its boundaries and be an active participant in policy development and implementation at the global level.

Spiritual care

Finally, one of the most important aspects in palliative care is being able to give attention to the spiritual needs of the person (child and adult), parents and families respectively. Personal beliefs about death and dying provide the person and family with the necessary strength to cope with what is known to be the most difficult period in one's life trajectory: facing death. This inner strength achieved through one's spirituality and personal beliefs can provide the most consistent source of comfort in a difficult time. Health care professionals, according to the guidelines propagated by the WHO (1998), need to acquaint themselves with the person's and family's spiritual beliefs when providing care. True spiritual care must be non-judgemental and respectful. In palliative care, one is challenged to find a way to achieve this aim without being too intrusive. The utmost of all aims is, naturally, to help the dying persons and families achieve a measure of peace.

Where do we go from here?

Similar to the approach used in Chapter 10, a number of recommendations for effective palliative care services are provided. These recommendations address clinical, educational, organisational and policy issues in palliative care and are applicable to both children and adults:

- Palliative care for children and adults should comprise a comprehensive approach focusing on physical, psychological, social, cultural and spiritual needs.
- An interdisciplinary multiprofessional approach is recommended and should be used.
- Palliative care can be effectively provided at home if the patient and family so wish.
- The use of clinical practice guidelines for the management of pain and other symptoms is advocated.
- It is recommended that the management of pain be based on the WHO guidelines for pain relief and palliative care.
- Misconceptions regarding opioids need to be corrected.
- The combination of pharmacological, supportive, physical and psychological therapies should be advocated in the relief of pain and other symptoms.
- Health care professionals should receive appropriate education and training in palliative care.
- Undergraduate and postgraduate teaching and certification systems for physicians and nurses should emphasise knowledge of palliative care.
- Evidence-based palliative care needs to have the foremost priority in the field.
- Research on effectiveness and efficiency of palliative care services continues to be important and warrants more attention in the future.
- The development of a national policy for service provision and funding should be possible.
- Palliative care should be an integral part of the national health care services in all countries.
- The allocation of funding in health care needs to be distributed evenly between curative and palliative services.
- Public awareness and public education should receive priority in palliative care.

References

Aaronson, N.K., Ahmedzai, S. & Bergman, B. (1993) The European Organisation for Research and Treatment of Cancer QLQ-C30: a quality of life instrument for use in international clinical trails in oncology. *Journal of Nat Cancer Institute*, **85**(5), 365–76.

Abma, T.A. (2000) Evaluating palliative care: facilitating reflexive dialogue about an ambiguous concept. *Medicine, Health Care & Philosophy*, 1, 1–16.

Abrahm, J. L., Callshan, J., Rosetti, K. & Pierre, L. (1996) The impact of a hospice consultation team on the care of veterans with advanced cancer. *Journal of Pain and Symptom Management*, 12, 23–31.

Abu-Saad, H. (1984) Assessing children's responses to pain. *Pain*, 19, 63–171.

Abu-Saad, H.H. (1989) Towards the development of an instrument to measure pain in children: Dutch study. *Advances in Pain Research & Therapy: Pediatric Pain*, pp. 101–107. Raven Press, New York.

Abu-Saad, H., Kroonen, E. & Halfens, R. (1990) On the development of a Dutch Pain Assessment Tool for Children. *Pain*, **43**(2), 249–56.

Abu-Saad, H.H. (1993) Nursing: the Science and the Practice. *International Journal of Nursing Studies*, 3, 287–94.

Abu-Saad. H.H. (1994) Pain in Children: developing a programme of research. *Disability and Rehabilitation*, **16**(1), 45–50.

Abu-Saad, H.H., Pool, H. & Tulkens, B. (1994) Further validity testing of the Abu-Saad Paediatric Pain Assessment Tool. *Journal of Advanced Nursing*, 19, 1063–71.

Abu-Saad, H.H. & Uiterwijk, M. (1995) Pain in Children with Juvenile Rheumatoid Arthritis: A Descriptive Study. *Pediatric Research*, **38** (2), 194–7.

ACT (1997) *Health guide to the development of children's palliative care services.* Association for Children with Life-threatening or Terminal Conditions and their Families, Royal College of Pediatrics and Child Health, London.

Addington-Hall, J.M., McDonald, L.D., Anderson, H.R. & Freeling, P. (1991) Dying from cancer: the views of bereaved family and friends about the experiences of terminally ill patients. *Palliative Medicine*, 5, 207–14.

Addington-Hall, J.M., McDonald, L.D., Anderson, H.R., Chamberlain, J., Freeling, P., Bland, J.M. & Raftery, J. (1992) Randomized controlled trial of effects of coordinating care for terminally ill cancer patients. *British Medical Journal*, 305, 1317–22.

Addington-Hall, J.M. & McCarthy, M. (1995a) Dying from cancer; results of a national population-based investigation. *Palliative Medicine*, 9, 295–305.

Addington-Hall, J.M. & McCarthy M. (1995b). Regional study of care for the dying: methods and sample characteristics. *Palliative Medicine*, 9, 27–35.

Ahmedzai, S. (1990) Measuring quality of life in hospice care. *Oncology*, **4**(5), 115–19.

Ahmedzai, S., Morton, A. & Reid, J. (1991) Quality of death in lung cancer: patients' reports and relatives' retrospective opinions. In *Psychosocial Oncology*, (eds M. Watson *et al.*). Pregnon Press, Oxford.

Ahmedzai, S. (1993a) Palliation of respiratory symptoms. In *The Oxford Textbook of Palliative Medicine*, (D. Doyle), pp. 349–78. Oxford University Press, London.

Ahmedzai, S. (1993b) The medicalization of dying: a doctor's view. In *The Future for Palliative Care*, (ed. D. Clark). Open University Press, Buckingham.

Ajemian, I. (1993) The interdisciplinary team. *Oxford Textbook of Palliative Medicine*, 1st edn, pp. 17–28). Oxford University Press, Oxford/New York/Tokyo.

Alter, C.L. (1996) Palliative and supportive care of patients with pancreatic cancer. *Seminars in Oncology*, 23(2), 229–40.

Arts, S.E., Huijer Abu-Saad H. & G.D. Champion (1994) Age-related response to Lidocaine-Prilocaine (EMLA) Emulsion and effect of music distraction on the pain of intravenous cannulation. *Pediatrics*, 93(5), 797–801.

Ashby, M. & Stoffell, B. (1991) Therapeutic ratio and defined phases: proposal of ethical framework for palliative care. *British Medical Journal*, 302(6788), 1322–4.

Axelsson, B. & Christensen, S.B. (1998) Evaluation of a hospital-based palliative support service with particular regard to financial outcome measures. *Palliative Medicine*, 12, 41–9.

Axelsson, B. & Sjoden, B.O. (1998) Assessment of quality of life in palliative care–psychometric properties of a short questionnaire. *Acta Oncologica*, 38(2), 229–37.

Baar F. (1999) Palliative care for the terminally ill in the Netherlands: the unique role of nursing homes. *European Journal of Palliative Care* 6(5), 169–172.

Babul, N. & Darke, A.C. (1993) Front line dispatch. *Journal of Palliative Care*, 9(4), 19–25.

Ballinx, M. (1995) Resultaten van een palliatief support thema in een algemeen ziekenhuis. *Verpleegkundigen en Gemeenschapszorg*, 51(3), 105–109.

Barakat, P.L., Sills, R. & LaBagnara, S. (1995) Management of fatal illness and death in children and their parents. *Pediatrics in Review*, 16(11), 419–23.

Barone, J.A., Jessen, L.M., Colaizzi, J.L. & Bierman, R.H. (1994) Cisapride: a gastrointestinal prokinetic drug. *Annal Pharmacotherapy*, 28, 488–99.

Barret, D. (1982) *World Christian Encyclopedia*. Oxford University Press, New York.

Barraclough J. (1997) ABC of palliative care, depression, anxiety and confusion. *British Medical Journal*, 315, 1365–8.

Baumann, T.J., Batenhorst, R.L., Graves, D.A., Foster, T.S. & Bennett, R.L. (1986) Patient-controlled analgesia in the terminally ill cancer patient. *Drug Intelligence and Clinical Pharmacy*, 20, 297–301.

Beller, E., Tattersall, M., Lunley, T., Levi, J. Dalley, D. *et al.* (1997) Improved quality of life with megestrol acetate in patients with endocrine-insensitive advanced cancer: a randomised controlled trial. *Annals of Oncology* 8, 277–83.

Bennegard, K., Eden, E., Ekman L., Schertsen, T. & Lundholm K. (1983) Metabolic response of whole body and peripheral tissues to enteral nutrition in weight-losing cancer and non-cancer patients. *Gastroenterology*, 85, 92–9.

Bertero, C.E. & Ek, A.C. (1993) Quality of life of adults with acute leukaemia. *Journal of Advanced Nursing*, 18, 1346–53.

Beyer, J. & Aradine, C. (1984) *The Oucher: a user's manual and technical report*. Judson, Evanston, Illinois.

Bierenbaum, H.G. & Kidder, D. (1984) What does hospice cost? *American Journal of Public Health*, 74, 689–97.

Bierenbaum, L.K. (1992) Terminal care costs in childhood cancer. *Pediatric Nursing*, 18(3), 285–8.

Bieri, D., Reeve, R.A., Champion, G.D., Addicoat, L. & Ziegler, J.B. (1990) The Faces Pain Scale for the self-assessment of the severity of pain experienced by children:

development, initial validation and preliminary investigation for ratio scale properties. *Pain*, 41, 39–150.

Bluebond-Langer, M. (1978) *The Private Worlds of Dying Children*. Princeton University Press, Princeton, NJ.

Blumhuber, H., de Conno, F. & Hanks, G.W. (1996) Report of the European Association for Palliative Care. *Journal of Pain and Symptom Management*, 12(2), 82–4.

Bly, J.L. & Kissinck, P. (1994) Hospice care for patients living alone: results of a demonstration program. *The Hospice Journal*, 9(4), 9–20.

Boekema, A.G., Mak, A.C.A., Wigboldus, A.M. & Wulferink, A. (1994) Pijnbestrijding bij kanker: een knelpunetenanalyse (Pain management in cancer; an analysis). *Medisch Contact*, 49(4), 128–31.

Boersma, F.P., Noorduin, H. & van de Bussche, G. (1989) Epidural Sufentanil for cancer pain control in outpatients. *Regional Anesthesia*, (November–December), 293–7.

Boisvert, M.C. & Cohen, S.R. (1995) Opioid use in advanced malignant disease: why do different centers use vastly different doses? A plea for standardized reporting. *Journal of Pain and Symptom Management*, 10(8), 632–8.

Bonica, J. (1985) Treatment of cancer pain: current status and future needs. In *Advances in Pain Research and Therapy* (ed. H.L. Fields). Raven Press, New York.

Bouffet, E., Zucchinelli, V., Blanchard, P., Costanzo, P., Frappaz, D. & Roussin, G. (1996) La scolarite en fin de vie. Quels objectifs, quel espoir? *Archives of Pediatrics*, (3), 555–60.

Boyd, K.J. (1992) The working patterns of hospice based home care teams. *Palliative Medicine*, 6, 131–9.

Boyd, K.J. (1994) Hospice home care in the United Kingdom. *Annals of Academic Medicine*, Singapore, 23(2), 271–4.

Boyd, K.J., & Kelly, M. (1997) Oral morphine as symptomatic treatment of dyspnea in patients with advanced cancer. *Palliative Medicine*, 11, 277–81.

Bradley, B., Mogg, K. & Millar, N. (1996) Implicit memory bias in clinical and non-clinical depression. *Behavioural Research Therapy*, 34(12), 865–79.

Brady, M.J. & Cella, D. (1999) Assessing quality of life in palliative care. *Cancer Treatment and Research*, 100, 203–16.

Breitbart, W. & Jacobsen, P.B. (1996) Psychiatric symptom management in terminal care. *Clinics in Geriatric Medicine*, 12(2), 329–47.

Brooks, C.H. & Smyth Staruch, K. (1984) Hospice home care cost savings to third-party insurers. *Medical Care*, 22(8), 691–703.

Bruera, E., Fox, R. & Chadwick, S. (1987) Changing pattern in the treatment of pain and other symptoms in advanced cancer patients. *Journal of Pain and Symptom Management*, 2, 139–45.

Bruera, E., McMillan, K., Kuehn, N. *et al.* (1990) A controlled trial of megestrol acetate on appetite, caloric intake, nutritional status and other symptoms in patients with advanced cancer. *Cancer*, 66, 1279–82.

Bruera, E., Kuehn N. & Miller, M.J. (1991) The Edmonton Symptom Assessment System (ESAS); a simple method for the assessment of palliative care patients. *Journal of Palliative Care*, 7(2), 6–9.

Bruera, E., de Stoutz, N., Velasco-Leiva, A., Schoeller, T. & Hanson, J. (1993) Effects of oxygen on dyspnea in hypoxemic terminal cancer patients. *Lancet*, 342(8862), 13–14.

Bruera, E., McEachern, T.J., Spachynski, K.A., Le Gatt, D.F., McDonald, R.N., Babul, N., Harsanyi, Z. & Darke, A.C. (1994a) Comparison of the efficacy, safety, and pharmacokinetics of controlled release and immediate release metoclopromide for the management of chronic nausea in patients with advanced cancer. *Cancer*, 74, 3204–11.

Bruera, E., Suarez-Almazor, M., Velasco, A. & Bertolino, M. (1994b), The assessment of constipation in terminal cancer patients admitted to a palliative care unit: a retrospective review. *Journal of Pain Symptom Management*, 9, 515–19.

Bruera, E. (1996) Quality assurance in palliative care – a growing 'must'? (editorial comment). *Support Care Cancer*, 4(3), 1.

Bruera, E. & Neumann, C.M. (1998) Management of specific symptom complexes in patients receiving palliative care. *Journal of Canadian Medical Association*, 158(13), 1717–26.

Bruera, E., Neumann, C., Pituskin, E., Calder, K. *et al.* (1999) Thalidomide in patients with cachexia due to terminal cancer: preliminary report. *Annals of Oncology*, 10, 857–9.

Bruntink, R. (1998) Nursing homes in palliative care, (Verpleeghuizen profileren zich op palliatieve zorg). *Pallium, Journal of Palliative Care, (Pallium Tijdschrift voor Palliatieve Zorg)*, 1(1), 9–13.

Bukberg J., Perman D. & Holland, J.C. (1984) Depression in hospitalised cancer patients, *Psychsomatic Medicine*, 46(3), 199–212.

Burdon, J., Juniper, E.F., Kilian, F., Hargreave, F.E. & Campbell, E.J.M. (1992) The perception of breathlessness in asthma. *American Review of Respiratory Disease*, 126, 825–8.

Burne, R. & Hunt, A. (1987) Use of opiates in terminally ill children. *Palliative Medicine*, 1, 27–30.

Burucoa, B. (1991) Palliative care: definition and structure. *Bulletin Cancer*, 78(4), 393–4.

Butters, E., Higginson, I., George, R., Smits, A. & McArthy, M. (1992) Assessing the symptoms, anxiety, and practical needs of HIV/AIDS patients receiving palliative care. *Quality of Life Research*, 1, 47–51.

Butters, E., Higginson, I., George, R. & McCarthy. M. (1993) Palliative care of people with HIV/AIDS: views of patients, carers, and providers. *AIDS Care*, 5, 105–16.

Byock, I.R. (1994) Ethics from a hospice perspective. *American Journal of Hospital Palliative Care*, 11(4), 9–11.

Campbell, M.L. (1996) Program assessment through outcomes analysis: efficacy of a comprehensive supportive care team for end-of-life-care. *AACN Clinical Issues*, 7(1), 159–67.

Caraceni, A., Cherny, N., Fainsinger, R., Kaasa, S., Poulain, P., Radbruch, L, & De Conno, F. (2000) Pain measurement tools and methods in clinical research in palliative care: recommendations of an expert working group of the European Association of Palliative Care. *Journal of Pain and Symptom Management,* (in press).

Carlson, P., Simacek, M., Henry, W., & Martinson, I.M. (1985) A model home care program for the dying child. *Issues in Comprehensive Pediatric Nursing*, 8(1–6), 113–27.

Carlson, R.W., Devich, L. & Frank, R.R. (1988) Development of a comprehensive supportive care team for the hopelessly ill on a university medical service. *Journal of American Medical Association*, 259(3), 378–83.

Cartwright, A. & Seale, C. (1990) *The natural history of a survey: an account of the methodological issues encountered in a study of life before death.* King Edwards Hospital Fund for London, London.

Cassel, E. (1991) *The nature of suffering and the goals of medicine.* Oxford University Press, New York.

Castle, N.G., Mor, V., & Banszak, J.B. (1997) Special care hospice units in nursing homes. *The Hospice Journal*, 12(3), 59–69.

Centeno-Cortes, C. & Nunez-Olante, J.M. (1994) Questioning diagnosis disclosure in terminal cancer patients: a prospective study evaluating patients' responses. *Palliative Medicine*, 8, 39–44.

Chambers, E.J. & Oakhill, A. (1995) Models of care for children dying of malignant disease. *Palliative Medicine*, 9(13), 181–5.

Chan, A.W. & Woodruff, R.K. (1991) Palliative care in a general teaching hospital. *The Medical Journal of Australia*, 155(4), 597–8.

Chochinov, H.M., Wilson, K.G., Enns, M. & Lander, S. (1994) Prevalence of depression in the terminally ill: Effects of diagnostic criteria and symptom threshold judgements. *American Journal of Psychiatry*, 151(4), 537–40.

Chochinov, H.M., Wilson, K.G., Enns, M. *et al.* (1995) Desire for death in the terminally ill. *American Journal of Psychiatry*, 152, 1185–91.

Chochinov, H.M., Wilson, K.G., Enns, M. & Lander, S. (1997) Are you depressed. Screening for depression in the terminally ill. *American Journal of Psychiatry*, 154, 674–6.

Chochinov, H.M., Wilson, K., Enns, M. & Lander, S. (1998) Depression, hopelessness and suicidal ideation in the terminally ill. *Psychosomatics*, 39(4), 366–9.

Clark, D. & Seymour, J. (1999) *Reflections on Palliative Care*. Open University Press, Buckingham.

Cleeland, C.S., Gonin, R., Hatfield, A.K., Edmonson, J.H., Blum, R.H., Stewart, J.H. & Pandya, K.J. (1994) Pain and its treatment in outpatients with metastatic cancer. *New England Journal of Medicine*, 330, 592–6.

Cleeland, C.S., Nakamura, Y., Mendoza, T.R., Edwards, K.R., Douglas, J. & Serlin, R.C. (1996) Dimensions of the impact of cancer in a four country sample: new information from multidimensional scaling. *Pain*, 67, 267–73.

Cohen, K. (1979) Hospice, prescription for terminal care. Aspen Systems Corporation, Germantown, Maryland/London.

Cohen, S.R., Balfour, M.M., Strobel, M.G. & Bui, F. (1995) The McGill quality of life questionnaire: a measure of quality of life appropriate for people with advanced disease. A preliminary study of validity and acceptability. *Palliative Medicine*, 9, 207–19.

Cohen, S.R., Mount, B., Bruera, E. & Provost, M. (1997) Validity of the McGill quality of life questionnaire in the palliative setting: a multi-center Canadian study demonstrating the importance of the extestential domain. *Palliative Medicine*, 11, 3–20.

Collins, J.J., Grier, H.E., Kinney, H.C. & Berde, C.B. (1995) Control of severe pain in children with terminal malignancy. *The Journal of Pediatrics*, 126, 653–7.

Collins, J.S. (1996) Intractable pain in children with terminal cancer. *Journal of Palliative Care*, 12(3), 29–34.

Collins, J.J., Stevens, M.M. & Cousens, P. (1998) Home care for the dying child; A parent's perception. *Australian Family Physician*, 27(7), 610–14.

Collins, J.J., Dunkel, I.J., Gupta, S. K., Inturrissi, C. E., Lapin, J., Palmer, L.N., Weinstein, S.M. & Portenoy, R.K. (1999) Transdermal fentanyl in children with cancer pain: feasibility, tolerability, and pharmacokinetic correlates. *The Journal of Pediatrics*, 134(3), 319–23.

Conill, C., Verger, E., Henriques, I, Saiz, N. *et al.* (1997) Symptom prevalence in the last week of life. *Journal of Pain and Symptom Management*, 14(6), 328–31.

Connolly, M. (1994) Palliative care. Partners in care. *Nursing Times*, 90(44), 58–61.

Constantini, M., Camoirano, E., Maddedu, L., Bruzzi, P., Verganelli, E. & Henriquet, F. (1993) Palliative home care and place of death among cancer patients: a population based study. *Palliative Medicine*, 7, 323–31.

Conte, P.M., Walco, G.A., Sterling, C.M., Engel, R.G. & Kuppenheimer, W.G. (1999) Procedural pain management in pediatric oncology: a review of the literature. *Cancer Investigation*, 17(6), 448–59.

COPZ (1998) Centra voor Ontwikkeling van Palliatieve Zorg in de terminale fase. Centers for the development of palliative care, Den Haag, The Netherlands.

Cornaglia, C., Massino, L. & Haupt, R. (1984) Incidence of pain in children with neoplastic diseases. *Pain*, 2(Suppl.), 28.

Corner, J., Planth, H., Hern, R. & Bailey, C. (1996) Non-pharmacological interventions for breathlessness in lung cancer. *Palliative Medicine*, 10(4), 299–305.

Corr, C.A. & Corr, D.M. (1985) Pediatric hospice care. *Pediatrics*, 76(5), 775–80.

Coughlan, M.C. (1993) Knowledge of diagnosis, treatment and its side-effects in patients receiving chemotherapy for cancer. *European Journal for Cancer Care*, 2, 66–71.

Coyle, N., Adelhardt, J., Foley, K. & Portnenoy, K. (1990) Character of terminal illness in the advanced cancer patient: Pain and other symptoms during the last four weeks of life. *Journal of Pain and Symptom Management*, 5(2), 83–93.

Coyle, N. (1997) Interdisciplinary collaboration in hospital palliative care: chimera or goal (editorial). *Palliative Medicine*, 11, 265–6.

Cuijk van, A. (1996) *Bruikbaarheid en betrouwbaarheid van het supportive team assessment schedule (Validity and reliability of the supportive team assessment schedule)*. Doctoraalscriptie (Masters thesis), Faculty of Health Sciences, Maastricht University, Maastricht.

Culpepper-Morgan, J.A., Inturrisi, C.E., Portenoy, R.K. *et al.* (1992) Treatment of opiod-induced constipation with oral naloxone: a pilot study. *Clinical Pharmacological Therapy* 52, 90–95.

Curtis, S. (1986) The effect of music on pain relief and relaxation in the terminally ill. *Journal of Music Therapy*, 23(1), 10–14.

Curtis, A.E & Fernsler, J.I. (1989) Quality of life of oncology hospice patients: A comparison of patients and primary caregiver reports. *Oncology Nursing Forum*, 16(91), 49–53.

Dangel, T., Fowler-Kerry, S., Karwacki, M. & Bereda, J. (2000) An evaluation of a home palliative care program for children. *Ambulatory Child Health*, 6(2), 110–14.

Davies, B. & Oberle, K. (1990) Dimensions of the supportive role of the nurse in palliative care. *Oncology Nursing Forum*, 17(1), 87–94.

Davies, B., Deveau, E., deVeber, B., Howell, D., Martinson, I., Papadatou, D., Pask, E. & Stevens, M. (1998) Experiences of mothers in five countries whose child died of cancer. *Cancer Nursing*, 21(5), 301–11.

De Conno, F., Caracenni, A., Groff, L., Brunelli, C., Donatti, I. & Ventafridda, V. (1996) Effect of home care on the place of death of advanced cancer patients. *European Journal of Cancer*, 32A(7), 1142–7.

Del Favero, A., Roila, F. & Tonato, M. (1993) Reducing chemotherapy-induced nausea and vomiting. Current perspectives and future possibilities. *Drug Safety*, 9, 410–28.

Derogatis, L.R., Morrow, G.R., Fetting, J., Penman D., Piasetsky, S., Schmale, A.M. *et al.* (1983) The prevalence of psychiatric disorders among cancer patients. *Journal of American Medical Association*, 249, 751–7.

Dessloch, A., Maiworm, M., Florin, I. & Schulze, C. (1992) Krankenhauspflege versus Hauskrankenpflege: Zur lebenqualitat bei terminalen tumorpatienten (Hospital nursing versus home care nursing: quality of life in terminal ill cancer patients). *Psychotherapy Psychosomatic Medicine Psychology*, 42, 424–9.

Devery K., Lennie I. & Cooney, N. (1999) Health outcomes for people who use palliative care services. *Journal of Palliative Care*, summer, 15(2), 5–12.

Dezube, B., Pardee, A., Chapman, B., Beckett, L. *et al.* (1993) Pentoxifylline decreases tumor necrosis factor expression and serum triglycerides in people with AIDS. *Journal of AIDS*, 6, 787–94.

Dicks, B. (1989) Palliative care. A vital cornerstone. *Nursing Times*, 85(44), 45–7.

Dobratz, M.C. (1990) Hospice nursing; present perspectives and future directives. *Cancer Nursing*, 13(2), 116–22.

Donabedian A. (1980) *The definition of quality and approaches to its assessment.* Health Administration Press, Michigan.

Donnelly S. & Walsh, D. (1995) The symptoms of advanced cancer. *Seminars in Oncology*, **22**(Suppl. 3), 67–72.

Dorrepaal, K.L. (1989) *Pijn bij Patienten met Kanker (Pain in Patients with Cancer).* Vrije Universiteit (Free University), Amsterdam.

Doyle, D., Hanks, G.W.C. & McDonald, N. (1993) *Oxford Textbook of Palliative Medicine.* Oxford University Press, Oxford.

Doyle, D. (1994) The future of palliative care. In *Dying, Death, & Bereavement: Theoretical Perspectives and Other Ways of Knowing*, (eds I.B. Corless, B.B. Germino & M. Pittman). Jone & Bartlett, Boston & London.

Doyle, D. H., Hanks, G.W.C. & MacDonald, N. (1998) *Oxford Textbook of Palliative Medicine*, 2nd edn. Oxford University Press, Oxford.

Duffy, C.M., Pollach, P., Levy, M., Budd, E., Caulfield, L. & Koren, G. (1990) Home based palliative care for children. *Palliative Care*, **6**(2), 8–114.

Dunlop, R.J. & Hockley, J.M. (1998) *Hospital-Based Palliative Care Teams: The Hospital-hospice Interface*, 2nd edn. Oxford University Press.

Dwyer, L. (1997) Palliative medicine in India. *Palliative Medicine*, **11**(6), 487–8.

Edmonds, P.L., Stuttaford, J.M., Penny, J., Lynch, A.M. & Chamberlain, J. (1998) Do hospital palliative care teams improve symptom control? Use of a modified STAS as an evaluation tool. *Palliative Medicine*, 12, 345–51.

Edwardson, S. (1983) The choice between hospital and home care for terminally ill children. *Nursing Research*, **32**(1), 29–34.

Ellenberg, L., Kellerman, J., Dash, J., Higgins, G. & Zeltzer, L. (1980) Use of hypnosis for multiple symptoms in an adolescent girl with leukaemia. *Journal of Adolescent Health Care*, 1, 132–6.

Ellershaw, J. (1995) Assessing the effectiveness of a hospital palliative care team. *Palliative Medicine*, 9, 145–52.

Elliott, S.C., Miser, A.W. & Dose, A.M. (1991) Epidemiologic features of pain in pediatric cancer patients; a co-operative community-based study. North Central Cancer Treatment Group and Mayo Clinic. *Clinical Journal of Pain*, **7**(4), 263–8.

Epstein, A., Hall, J., Tognotti, J., Son, L. & Conant, L. (1989) Using proxies to evaluate quality of life. *Medical Care*, **27**(3), 91–8.

Eynden van den, B. (1994) *Kwaliteit van leven in de palliatieve zorg (Quality of Life in Palliative Care).* Doctoraat proefscrift (PhD Dissertation), Universitaire Instelling Antwerpen (University of Antwerpen), Antwerp.

Fakhoury, W.K.H., McCarthy, M. & Addington-Hall, J. (1997) The effects of the clinical characteristics of dying cancer patients on informal caregivers' satisfaction with palliative care. *Palliative Medicine*, 11, 107–15.

Fakhoury, W.K.H. (1998) Satisfaction with palliative care: what should we be aware of? *International Journal of Nursing Studies*, 35, 171–6.

Farrell, M. & Sutherland, P. (1998) Providing paediatric palliative care: collaboration in practice. *Children's Nursing*, **7**(12), 712–16.

Ferrel, B.R., Johnston Taylor, E., Sattler, G.R., Fowler, M. & Cheyney, B.L. (1993) Searching for the meaning of pain; cancer patients', caregivers', and nurses' perspectives. *Cancer Practice*, 1, 185–94.

Field, D., Dand, P., Ahmedzai, S. & Biswas, B. (1992) Terminal illness: views of patients and their lay carers. *Palliative Medicine*, 6, 51–9.

Field, D. (1994) Client satisfaction with terminal care. *Progress in Palliative Care*, 2, 228–32.

Field, D.B., Devich, L.E. & Carlson, R.W. (1996) Impact of a comprehensive supportive care team on management of hopelessly ill patients with multiple organ failure. *Chest*, 2, 353–6.

Field, D., Hockey, J. & Small, N. (1997) *Death, Gender, & Ethnicity*. Routledge, London.

Filshie, J., Penn, K., Ashley, S. & Davis. C.L. (1996) Acupuncture in the relief of cancer-related breathlessness. *Palliative Medicine*, 10(2), 145–50.

Finlay I.G. & Dunlop, R. (1994) Quality of life assessment in palliative care. *Annals of Oncology*, Jan, 5(1), 13–18.

Finley, G.A. & McGrath, P.J. (eds) (1998) *Measurement of Pain in Infants and Children*. IASP Press, Seattle.

Folstein, M.F., Folstein, S.E. & McHugh, P.R. (1975) Mini-mental state. *Journal of Psychiatric Research*, 12, 189–98.

Francke, A.L., Persoon, A., Temmink D. & Kerkstra A. (1997) *Palliatieve Zorg in Nederland: een inventarisatiestudie naar palliatieve zorg, deskundigheidsbevordering en zorg voor zorgenden (Palliative Care in the Netherlands: An inventory into palliative care, professional development, and care of the carers)*. NIVEL, Nederlands Instituut voor Onderzoek van de Gezondheidszorg (Dutch Institute for Health Care Research), Utrecht.

Friel, P.B. (1982) Death and dying. *Annal of Internal Medicine*, 97(5), 767–71.

Gallagher, R.M. (1998) Chronic pain: a public health problem (editorial). *The Clinical Journal of Pain*, 14, 277–9.

Garland, E. (1994) Palliative care. Privileged position. *Nursing Times*, 90(44), 62–3.

Gauvain-Piquard, A, Rodary, C., Rezvani, A. & Serbouti, S. (1999) The development of the DEGRı a scale to assess pain in young children with cancer. *European Journal of Pain*, 3, 165–76.

George, R.J. (1991) Palliation in AIDS – where do we draw the line? (editorial). *Genitourinary Medicine*, 67(2), 85–6.

George, R.J. & Jennings, A.L. (1993) Palliative medicine. *Postgraduate Medical Journal*, 69(812), 429–49.

Gift, A.G. (1989) Validation of a vertical visual analogue scale as a measure of clinical dyspnoea. *Rehabilitation Nursing*, 14(6), 323–5.

Gift, A.G. (1990) Dyspnoea. *Nursing Clinics of North America*, 25(4), 955–65.

Give, C.W. & Stommel W. (1993) The influence of the cancer patient's symptoms. Functional status on patient's depression and family caregiver's reaction and depression. *Health Psychology*, 12, 277–85.

Glover, J., Dibble, S., Dodd, M.J. *et al.* (1995) Mood states of oncology outpatients: does pain make a difference? *Journal of Pain and Symptom Management*, 10, 120–28.

Goldberg, R.M., Loprinzi, C. & Mailliard, J. (1995) Pentoxifylline for treatment of cancer anorexia and cachexia. A randomised double blind placebo controlled trial. *Journal of Clinical Oncology*, 13, 2856–9.

Goldberg, R.J., Mor, V., Wiemann, M., Greer, D.S. & Hiris, J. (1986) Analgesic use in terminal cancer patients: report from the National Hospice study. *Journal of Chronic Disease*, 39(1), 37–45.

Goldin, G. (1981) A protohospice at the turn of the century: St. Luke's House, London, from 1893 to 1921. *Journal of History of Medical Allied Sciences*, 36(4), 383–415.

Goldman, A., Beardsmore, S. & Hunt, J. (1990) Palliative care for children with cancer–home, hospital, or hospice? *Archives of Diseases in Childhood*, 65, 641–3.

Goldman, A. (1990) The role of oral controlled-release morphine for pain relief in children with cancer. *Palliative Medicine*, 4, 279–85.

Goldman, A. (1992) Care of the dying child. In *Pediatric Oncology; Clinical Practice and*

Controversies, (eds P.N. Plowman & C.R. Pinkerton, pp. 618–29. Chapman & Hall Medical, London.

Goldman, A. (1994) *Care of the Dying Child*. Oxford University Press, Oxford.

Goldman, A. (1996) Home care of the dying child. *Journal of Palliative Care*, **12**(3), 16–19.

Goldman, A. (1998) ABC of palliative care; special problems of children. *British Medical Journal*, 316, 3 January, 49–52.

Goldstein, A. (1980) Thrills in response to music and other stimuli. *Physiological Psychology*, **8**(1), 126–9.

Graham, J., Ramirez, A.J., Cull, A., Finlay, I., Hoy, A. & Richards, M.A. (1996) Job stress and satisfaction among palliative care physicians. *Palliative Medicine*, 10, 185–94.

Grande, G.E., Barlay, S.I.G. & Todd, C.J. (1997a) Difficulty of symptom control and general practitioners' knowledge of patients' symptoms. *Palliative Medicine*, 11, 399–406.

Grande, G.E., Todd, C.J. & Barclay, S.I.G. (1997b) Support needs in the last year of life: patient and carer perspective. *Palliative Medicine*, 11, 202–208.

Grant M.M. & Rivera, L.M. (1995) Anorexia, cachexia and dysphagia: the symptom experience. *Seminars in Oncology Nursing*, **11**(4), 266–71.

Gray, A.J. & Elder, P. (1987) Hospice care, whose responsibility? *New Zealand Medical Journal*, **100**(835), 679–80.

Greer, D.S., Mor, V., Morris, J.N., Sherwood, S., Kidder, D. & Birnbaum, H. (1986) An alternative in terminal care: results of the National Hospice Study. *Journal of Chronic Diseases*, **39**(1), 9–26.

Grossman, S.A., Sheidler, V.R., Swedeen, K., Mucenski, J. & Piantadosi, S. (1991) Correlation of patient and care giver ratings of cancer pain. *Journal of Pain and Symptom Management*, 6, 53–7.

Guyatt, G.H., Berman, L.B., Townsend M., Pugsley, S. & Chambers L.W. (1987) A measure of quality of life for clinical trials in chronic lung disease. *Thorax*, 42, 773–8.

Guyatt, G.H., Keller, J.L., Jaeschke, R., Rosenbloom, D., Adachi, J.D. & Newhouse, M.T. (1990) The n-of-1 randomized clinical trial: clinical usefulness. *Annals of Internal Medicine*, 112, 293–9.

Hainsworth, J.D. (1993) Development of serotonin antagonists for the control of chemotherapy-induced emesis. *Seminars in Surgical Oncology*, 9, 279–84.

Hann, D.M., Jacobsen, P.B, Azzarello, L.M., Martin, S.C., Curran, S.L., Fields, K.K., Greenberg, H. & Lyman, G. (1998) Measurement of fatigue in cancer patients: developments and validation of the Fatigue Symptom Inventory. *Quality of Life Research*, 7, 301–10.

Hatcliff, S., Smith, P. & Daw, R. (1996) District nurses' perceptions of palliative care at home. *Nursing Times*, **92**(41), 36–7.

Hearn, J. & Higginson, I.J. (1997) Outcome measures in palliative care for advanced patients: a review. *Journal of Public Health Medicine*, **19**(2), 193–9.

Hearn, J.H. & Higginson, I.J. (1998) Do specialist palliative care teams improve outcomes for cancer patients? A systematic literature review. *Palliative Medicine*, 12, 317–32.

Hearn, J. & Higginson, I.J. (1999) Development and validation of a core outcome measure for palliative care: the palliative care outcome scale. *Quality in Health Care*, 8, 219–27.

Herth, K. (1993) Hope in the family caregiver of terminally ill people. *Journal of Advanced Nursing*, 18, 538–48.

Hewitt, M., McQuade, B. & Stevens, R. (1993) The efficacy and safety of ondansetron in the prophylaxis of cancer-chemotherapy induced nausea and vomiting in children. *Clinical Oncology*, 5, 11–14.

Heyse-Moore, L. (1991) Respiratory symptoms. In *The Management of Terminal Malignant Disease*, (C. Saunders & N. Sykes), pp. 76–93. Edward Arnold, London.

Higginson, I.J., Wade, A. & McCarthy, M. (1990) Palliative care: views of patients and their families. *British Medical Journal*, 301, 277–81.

Higginson, I.J., Wade, A. & McCarthy, M. (1992) Effectiveness of two palliative support teams. *Journal of Public Health Medicine*, 14, 50–56.

Higginson, I. J. (1993) Palliative care: a review of past changes and future trends. *Public Health Medicine*, 15(1), 3–8.

Higginson, I.J. & McCarthy, M. (1993) Validity of the support team assessment schedule: do staff's ratings reflect those made by patients and their families? *Palliative Medicine*, 7, 219–28.

Higginson, I. J. & Hearn, J. (1997) A multicenter evaluation of cancer pain control by palliative care teams. *Journal of Pain and Symptom Management*, 14, 29–35.

Hill, F. & Oliver, C. (1984) Hospice, the cost of in-patient care. *Health Trends*, 16, 9–11.

Hill, F. & Oliver, C. (1989) Hospice, an update on the cost of patient care. *Palliative Medicine*, 3, 119–24.

Hinton, J. (1979) Comparison of places and policies for terminal care. *Lancet*, 1, 29–32.

Hinton, J. (1996) Services given and help perceived during home care for terminal cancer. *Palliative Medicine*, 10, 125–34.

Hiraga, K., Mizugechi, T. & Takeda, F. (1991) The incidence of cancer pain and improvement of pain management in Japan. *Postgraduate Medical Journal*, 67 (suppl. 2), 314–25.

Holford, J.M. (1973) Terminal care. *Nursing Times*, 69(4), 113–15.

Holland, J.C., Morrow G. & Schmale, A. (1988) Reduction of anxiety and depression in cancer patients by alprazolam or by a behavioral technique. *Proceedings of the American Society of Clinical Oncology*, 6, 258.

Howarth, G. & Jefferys, M. (1996) Euthanasia: sociological perspectives. *British Medical Bulletin*, 52, 376–85.

Hughes, S.L., Cunnings, J. & Weaver, F. (1992) A randomised trial of the cost-effectiveness of VA hospital-based home care for the terminally ill. *Health Services Research*, 26, 801–17.

Humbert, N. (1997) Soins palliatiefs et pediatrie entre l'abondon et l'achamement (Palliative care in children; between abandonment and attachment). Revue Medicale Suisse Romande, 117(3), 197–200.

Hunt, A. (1990) A survey of signs, symptoms and symptom control in 30 terminally ill children. *Developmental Medicine and Child Neurology*, 32, 341–6.

Hunt, M. (1991) The identification and provision of care for the terminally ill at home by family members. *Sociology of Health and Illness*, 13, 375–95.

Hunt, A.B. & Burne, R. (1995) Medical and nursing problems of children with neuro-degenerative disease. *Palliative Medicine*, 9, 19–26.

Hunt, J.A. (1996) *Pediatric Oncology Outreach Nurse Specialists: The Impact of Funding Arrangements on their Professional Relationships*. Royal College of Nursing, London.

Hunt, A., Joel, S., Dick, G. & Goldman, A. (1999) Population pharmacokinetics of oral morphine and its glucuronides in children receiving morphine as immediate-release liquid or sustained-release tablets for cancer pain. *The Journal of Pediatrics*, 135(1), 47–55.

Ingham, J.M. & Protenoy, R.K. (1996) Symptom assessment. *Palliative Care*, 10, 21–39.

Irvine, D., Vincent L., Graydon, J.E., Bubela N. & Thopson L. (1994) The prevalence and correlates of fatigue in patients receiving treatment with chemotherapy and radio-therapy. *Cancer Nursing*, 5, 367.

James, L. & Johnson, B. (1997) The needs of parents of pediatric oncology patients during the palliative care phase. *Journal of Pediatric Oncology Nursing,* **14**(2), 83–95.

Jeffrey D. (1995) Appropriate palliative care: when does it begin. *European Journal of Cancer Care,* 4, 122–6.

Johnston, G. & Abraham, C. (1995) The WHO objectives for palliative care: to what extent are we achieving them? *Palliative Medicine,* **9**(2), 123–7.

Joisy, S.K. (1999) *Palliative Medicine Secrets.* Hanley & Belfus, Philadelphia.

Jones, R.V.H., Hansford, J. & Fiske, J. (1993) Death from cancer at home: the carer's perspective. *British Medical Journal,* (306), 249–51.

Jones, R.V.H. (1993) Teams and terminal cancer care at home: do patients and carers benefit? *Journal of Interprofessional Care,* (7), 239–45.

Kaasa S., Malt U., Hagen S., Wist E. & Moum, T. (1993) Psychological distress in cancer patients with advanced cancer. *Radiotherapeutic Oncology,* 27, 193–7.

Kaasa, S., Bjordal K. & Aaronson, N. (1995) The EORTC Core quality of life questionnaire: validity and reliability when analysed with patients treated with palliative radiotherapy. *European Journal of Cancer,* **31**a(13/14), 2260–63.

Kaasa, T., Loomis, J., Gilles, K., Bruera, E. & Hanson, J. (1997) The Edmonton Functional Assessment Tool: Preliminary Development and Evaluation for Use in Palliative Care. *Journal of Pain and Symptom Management,* **13**(1), 10–19.

Kaasa, S., Loge, J.H., Knobel, H., Jordhoy, S. & Brenne, E. (1999) Fatigue. Measures and relation to pain. *Acta Anesthesiol Scandinavica,* 939–47.

Kane, R.L., Wales, J., Bernstein, L., Leibowitz, A. & Kaplan, S. (1984) A randomised controlled trial of hospice care. *Lancet,* **1**(8382), 890–4.

Kane, R., Klein, S.J., Bernstein, L. & Rothenberg, R. (1985a) Hospice role in alleviating the emotional stress of terminal patients and their families. *Medical Care,* 23, 189–97.

Kane, R.L., Bernstein, L., Wales, J. & Rothenberg, R. (1985b) Hospice effectiveness in controlling pain. *Journal of American Medical Association,* 253, 2683–6.

Kane, R., Klein, S.J., Bernstein, L. & Rothenberg, R. (1986) The role of hospice in reducing the impact of bereavement. *Journal of Chronic Disease,* 39, 735–42.

Kearney, M. (1996) *Mortally Wounded.* Marino, Dublin.

Keating, S.B. (1996) Hospice care and its relationship to home care services: a case study. *Geriatric Nursing,* **17**(1), 41–3.

Keay, T.J. & Schonwetter, R.S. (1998) Hospice Care in the Nursing Home. *American Family Physician,* **57**(3), 491–4.

Kellerhear, A. (1990) *Dying of Cancer. The Final Years of Life.* Harwood Academic, Reading, Paris, Philadelphia.

Kindlen, M. (1988) Hospice home care services: a Scottish perspective. *Palliative Medicine,* 2, 115–21.

King, M., Lapsley, I., Llewellyn, S. & Tierney, A. (1993) Palliative Care: Availability and cost implications. *Health Bulletin,* 51, 370–84.

Klaschik, E. & Husebo, S. (1997) Palliative medicine. *Anaesthesist,* **46**(3), 177–85.

Klein, S. & Koretz, R.L. (1994) Nutrition support in patients with cancer. What do the data really show? *Nutrition in Clinical Practice,* 9, 91–100.

Kohler, J.A. & Radford, M. (1985) Terminal care for children dying of cancer: quantity and quality of life. *British Medical Journal,* **291**(7), 115–16.

Kopecky, E.A., Jacobson, S., Joshi, P., Martin, M. & Koren, G. (1997) Review of a home-based palliative care program for children with malignant and non-malignant diseases. *Journal of Palliative Care,* **13**(4), 28–33.

Kreitler, S., Chaitchik, S., Rapoport, Y., Kreitler, H. & Algor, R. (1993) Life satisfaction and health in cancer patients, orthopedic patients and healthy individuals. *Social Science and Medicine*, **36**(4), 547–56.

Kristjanson, L.J., Sloan, J.A., Dudgeon, D. & Adaskin, E. (1996) Family members' perceptions of palliative cancer care: predictors of family functioning and family members' health. *Journal of Palliative Care*, **12**, 10–20.

Krupp, L.B., Larva, N.G., Muir-Nasch, J. & Steinberg, A.D. (1989) The fatigue severity scale. Application to patients with multiple sclerosis and systemic lupus erythematosus. *Archives of Neurology*, **46**(10), 1121–3.

Kuuppelomaki, M. & Lauri, S. (1998) Cancer patients' reported experiences of suffering. *Cancer Nursing*, **21**(5), 364–9.

Lauer, M.E., Mulhern, R.K., Hoffman, G. & Camitta, B.M. (1986) Utilisation of home care in pediatric oncology: a national survey. *Cancer Nursing*, **9**, 102–107.

Laviano, A. & Meguid, M.M. (1996) Nutritional issues in cancer management. *Nutrition*, **12**, 358–71.

LeBaron, S. & Zeltzer, L.K. (1985) The role of imagery in the treatment of dying children and adolescents. *Developmental and Behavioral Pediatrics*, **6**(5), 252–8.

LeBaron, S., Zelzer, L.K., LeBaron, C., Scott, S.E. & Zelzer, P.M. (1988) Chemotherapy side-effects in pediatric oncology patients: drugs, age, and sex as risk factors. *Medical Pediatric Oncology*, **49**, 269–70.

Le Fevre, P., Devereux, J., Smith, S., Lawrie, S.M. & Cornbleet, M. (1999) Screening for psychiatric illness in the palliative care inpatient setting: a comparison between the Hospital Anxiety and Depression Scale and the General Health Questionnaire – 12. *Palliative Medicine*, **13**, 399–407.

Leff, S.L. (1956) *From Witchcraft to Worldhealth*. Lawrence & Wishart, London.

Leland, J.Y. & Schonwetter, R.S. (1997) Advances in hospice care. *Clinical Geriatric Medicine*, **13**(2), 381–401.

Levy, M.H. (1996) Pharmacological treatment of cancer pain. *New England Journal of Medicine*, **335**, 1124–32.

Liben, S. (1998) Home care for children with life-threatening illness. *Journal of Palliative Care*, **14**(3), 33–8.

Lindley, C.M., Hirsch, J.D., O'Neill, C.V., Transau, M.C., Gilbert, C.S. & Osterhaus, J.T. (1992) Quality of life consequences of chemotherapy-induced emesis. *Quality of Life Research*, **1**, 331–40.

Lloyd-Williams, M., Friedman, T. & Rudd, N. (1999) A survey of antidepressant prescribing in the terminally ill. *Palliative Medicine*, **13**, 243–8.

Lobchuk, M.M., Christjanson, L., Degner, L., Blood, P. & Sloan, J.A. (1997) Congruence between patients and primary family care givers. *Journal of Pain and Symptom Management*, **14**, 136–46.

Loprinzi, C.L., Ellison, N.M. & Schaid, D.J. (1990) Controlled trial of megestrol acetate for the treatment of cancer anorexia and cachexia. *Journal of National Cancer Institute*, **82**, 1127–32.

Lowe, J.H. (1981) *Interdisciplinary team* (HRA 81-27). US Department of Health and Human Services Publication, Washington.

Luczak, J. (1993) Palliative/hospice care in Poland. *Palliative Medicine*, **7**(1), 67–75.

Lunt, B.N. & Neale, C. (1987) A comparison of hospice and hospital. *Palliative Medicine*, **1**, 136–48.

Lynch, M. (1995) The assessment and prevalence of affective disorders in advanced cancer. *Journal of Palliative Care*, **11**(1), 10–18.

Maddocks, I. (1993) Australian and New Zealand Society of Palliative Medicine (letter). *Medical Journal of Australia*, **159**(1), 72.

Mah, M.A. & Johnston, C. (1993) Concerns of families in which one member has head and neck cancer. *Cancer Nursing*, 16, 382–7.

Maher, E.J., Mackenzie, C, Young, T. & Marks, D. (1996) The use of the Hospital Anxiety and Depression Scale (HADS) and the EORTC L-C30 questionnaires to screen for treatable unmet needs in patients attending routinely for radiotherapy. *Cancer Treatment Review*, 22 (Suppl A), 123–9.

Maltoni, M., Pirovano, M., Nanni, O., Labianca, R. & Amadori, D. (1994) Prognostic factors in terminal cancer patients. *European Journal of Palliative Care*, 1, 122–5.

Maltoni, M., Pirovano, M. & Scarpi, E. (1995) Prediction of survival of patients terminally ill with cancer. *Cancer*, 75, 2613–22.

Mancini, I. & Bruera, E. (1998) Constipation in advanced cancer patients. *Support Care Cancer*, 6, 356–64.

Martinson, I.M., Geis, D., Anglim, M., Petersch, E., Nesbit, M. & Kersey, J. (1977) Home care for the child. *American Journal of Nursing*, 11, 1815–17.

Martinson, I.M., Armstrong, G.C. & Geis. D.P. (1978) Home care for children dying of cancer. *Pediatrics*, 62, 106–13.

Martinson, I.M. & Martinson, P. (1983) *Developing Theory from Practice*. C.V. Mosby, St. Louis.

Martinson, I.M., Moldow, D.G. & Armstrong, G.D. (1986) Home care for children dying of cancer. *Research in Nursing and Health*, 9, 11–16.

Martinson, I. (1996) An international perspective on palliative care for children. *Journal of Palliative Care*, 12(3), 13–15.

Masera, G., Spinetta, J.J., Jankovic, M., Ablin, A., D'Angio, G.J., van Dongen-Melman, J., Eden, T., Martins, A., Mulhern, R.K., Oppenheim, D., Topf, R. & Chesler, M.A. (1999) Guidelines for assistance to terminally ill children with cancer: a report of the SIOP (International Society of Paediatric Oncology) working committee on psychosocial issues in pediatric oncology. *Medical and Pediatric Oncology*, 32, 44–48.

Massie, M.J., Holland, J.C. & Straker, N. (1989) Psychotherapeutic interventions. In *Handbook of Psychooncology: Psychosocial Care of the Patient with Cancer*, (J.C. Holland *et al.*). Oxford University Press, New York.

Massie, M.J. & Holland, J.C. (1990) Depression and the cancer patient. *Journal of Clinical Psychiatry*, 51, 12–17.

Max, M.B. (1990) Improving outcomes of analgesic treatment: is education enough? *Annals of Internal Medicine*, 113, 885–9.

McCaffery, M. (1992) Pain control; barriers to use of available information. *Cancer*, 14, 38–49.

McCalum, R.W. (1991) Cisapride: a new class of prokinetic agent. *American Journal of Gastroenterology*, 86, 135–49.

McCord, M. & Cronin-Stubbs, D. (1992) Operationalising dyspnea: focus on measurement. *Heart & Lung*, 21, 167–79.

McCusker, J. & Stoddard, A.M. (1987) Effects of an expanding home care program. *Medical Care*, 25, 373–84.

McGrath, P.A. (1996) Development of the World Health Organisation Guidelines on Cancer Pain Relief and Palliative Care in Children. *Journal of Pain and Symptom Management*, 12(2), 87–92.

McGrath, P.J. (1996) Attitudes and beliefs about medication and pain management in children. *Journal of Palliative Care*, 12(3), 46–50.

McGrath, P.J. (1998) Behavioral measures of pain. In *Measurement of Pain Infants and Children*, (eds G.A. Finley & P.J. McGrath), vol 10, 83–102. IASP Press, Seattle.

McNair, D., Lorr, M. & Deoppleman, L.F. (1981) *Profile of Mood States Manual*. Educational and Industrial Testing Service, San Diego.

McNally, J.C., Bohnet, N.L. & Lindquist, M.E. (1996) Hospice nursing. *Seminars in Oncology Nursing*, **12**(3), 238–43.

McWhinney, I.R., Bass, M.J. & Donner, A. (1994) Evaluation of a palliative care service: problems and pitfalls. *British Medical Journal*, 309, 1340–42.

Melvin, T.A., Ozbek, I.N. & Eberle, D.E. (1995) Recognition of depression. *Hospice*, **10**(3), 39–46.

Mercadante, S., Dardanoni, G., Salvaggio, L., Armata, M.G. & Agnello A. (1997) Monotoring of opioid therapy. *Journal of Pain and Symptom Management*, **13**(4), 204–12.

Minagawa, H., Uchitomi, Y., Yamawaki, S. & Ishitani, K. (1996) Psychiatric morbidity in terminally ill cancer patients. *Cancer*, **78**(5), 1131–6.

Mino, J. (1999) Assessing the outcome of palliative care. *European Journal of Palliative Care*, **6**(6), 203–205.

Miser, A.W., McCalla, J. & Dothage, J.A. (1987a) Pain as a presenting symptom in children and young adults with malignancy. *Pain*, **29**(1), 85–90.

Miser, A.W., Dothage, J.A. & Wesley, R.A. (1987b) The prevalence of pain in a pediatric and young adult cancer population. *Pain*, **29**(1), 73–83.

Molassiotis, A., van den Akker, O.B.A., Milligan, D.W., Goldman, J.M. & Boughton, B.J. (1996) Psychological adaptation and symptom distress in bone marrow transplant recipients. *Psycho-oncology*, 5, 9–22.

Moldow, D.G., Henry, W. & Martinson, I.M. (1982) The cost of home care for dying children. *Medical Care*, 11, 1154–60.

Molen van der, B. (1995) Dyspnoea: a study of measurement instruments for the assessment of dyspnoea and the application for patients with advanced cancer. *Journal of Advanced Nursing*, 22, 948–56.

Mor, V., Wachtel, T.J. & Kidder, D. (1985) Patient predictors of hospice choice; hospice versus home care programs. *Medical Care*, **23**(9), 1115–19.

Mor, V. (1987) Cancer patients' quality of life over the disease course: lessons from the real world. *Journal of Chronic Disease*, **40**(6), 535–44.

Mor, V., Stalker, M.Z. & Gralla, R. (1988a) Day hospital as an alternative to inpatient care for cancer patients: a random assignment trial. *Journal of Clinical Epidemiology*, 41, 771–85.

Mor, V., Greer, D.S. & Kastenbaum, R. (1988b) *The Hospice Experiment*. Johns Hopkins University, Baltimore.

Morita, T, Tsunoda, J. & Inoue, S. (1999) Contributing factors to physical symptoms in terminally ill cancer patients. *Journal of Pain and Symptom Management*, **18**(5), 338–46.

Morris, J.N. & Sherwood, S. (1987) Quality of life of cancer patients at different stages in the disease trajectory. *Journal of Chronic Diseases*, 40, 545–53.

Morris, D. (1997) Palliation: shielding the patient from the assault of symptoms. *Academy Update*, **7**(3), 1–11. American Academy of Hospice and Palliative Medicine, Gainseville, Fl.

Mystakidou K., Befon, S., Liossi C. & Vlachos, L. (1998) Comparison of the efficacy and safety of tropisetron, metoclopramide and chlorpromazine in the treatment of emesis associated with advanced cancer. *Cancer*, **83**(6), 1214–23.

NCHSPCS (1995) *Specialist Palliative Care: A statement of definitions*. National Council for Hospice and Specialist Palliative Care Services, London.

Nekolaichuk, C. L., Bruera, E., Spachynski, K. & MacEachern, T. (1999) A comparison of patient and proxy symptom assessments in advanced cancer patients. *Palliative Medicine*, **13**(4), 311–23.

Ng K. & von Gunten C.F. (1998) Symptoms and attitudes of 100 consecutive patients admitted to an acute hospice/palliative care unit. *Journal of Pain and Symptom Management*, **16**(5), 307–16.

NHO (1993) *Standards of a hospice program of care*. National Hospice Organization, Arlington, Virginia.

Oberst, M.T., Thomas S.E., Gass, K.A. & Ward, S.E. (1989) Care giving demands and appraisal of stress among family caregivers. *Cancer Nursing*, 12, 209–15.

O'Neill, B. & Rodway, A. (1998) ABC of palliative care. Care in the community. *British Medical Journal*, **316**(7128), 373–7.

Parkes, C.M. (1979) Terminal care: evaluation of an inpatient service at St Christopher's Hospice. *Postgraduate Medical Journal*, 55, 517–22.

Parkes, C.M. (1980) Terminal care: evaluation of an advisory domiciliary service at St Christopher's Hospice. *Postgraduate Medical Journal*, 56, 685–9.

Parkes, C.M. (1984) Hospice versus hospital care – re-evaluation after 10 years as seen by surviving spouses. *Postgraduate Medical Journal*, 60, 12–24.

Parkes, C.M. (1985) Terminal care: home, hospital, or hospice. *Lancet*, 1, 155–7.

Passik, S.D. & Cooper, M. (1999) Complicated delirium in a cancer patient successfully treated with olanzapine. *Journal of Pain and Symptom Management*, **17**(3), 219–23.

Payne, S. (1992) A study of quality of life in cancer patients receiving palliative chemotherapy. *Social Science and Medicine*, **35**(12), 1505–1509.

Payne, S. (1998) Depression in palliative care patients: a literature review. *International Journal of Palliative Nursing*, **4**(4), 184–91.

Perakyla, A. (1989) Appealing to the experience of the patient in the care of the dying. *Sociology of Health and Illness*, 11, 117–34.

Peruselli, C., Paci, E., Franceschi, P., Legori, T. & Mannucci, F. (1997) Outcome evaluation in a home palliative care service. *Journal of Pain and Symptom Management*, **13**(3), 158–65.

Phipps, W. (1988) The origin of hospices/hospitals. *Death Studies*, vol. 12, pp. 91–9, Hemisphere Publishing Corporation.

Piper, B.F., Rieger, P.T., Brophy, L. *et al.* (1989) Recent advances in the management of biotherapy side-effects: fatigue. *Oncol Nursing Forum*, 16, 27–34.

Piper, B. F. (1993) Fatigue. In *Pathophysiological Phenomenon in Nursing; Human Responses to Illness*, (eds V. Carrieri-Kohlman, A.M. Lindsey & C.M. West). WB Saunders, Philadelphia.

Plumb, J.D. & Ogle, K.S. (1992) Hospice care. *Primary Care*, **19**(4), 807–20.

Portenoy, R.K. (1996) Opioid therapy for chronic non-malignant pain: a review of the critical issues. *Journal of Pain and Symptom Management*, **11**(4), 203–17.

Pratheepawanit, N., Salek, M.S. & Finlay, I.G. (1999) The applicability of quality of life assessment in palliative care: comparing two quality of life measures. *Palliative Medicine*, 13, 325–34.

Raftery, J.P., Addington-Hall, J.M., MacDonald, L.D. & Anderson, H.R. (1996) A randomised controlled trial of the cost-effectiveness of a district coordinating service for terminally ill cancer patients. *Palliative Medicine*, 10, 151–6.

Raudonis, B.M. (1993) The meaning and impact of empathic relationships in hospice nursing. *Cancer Nursing*, 16, 304–9.

Reuben, D.B., Mor, V. & Hiris, J. (1988) Clinical symptoms and length of survival in patients with terminal cancer. *Archives of Internal Medicine*, 148, 1586–91.

Reuben, D.B. & Mor V. (1987) Dyspnoea in terminally ill cancer patients. *Chest*, 89(2), 234–6.

Rhoten, D. (1982) Fatigue and the post-surgical patient. In: *Concept Clarification in Nursing* (ed. E. Norris). Aspen Publishers Inc, Rockville, MD.

Rhymes, J.A. (1991) Home hospice care. *Clinics in Geriatric Medicine*, 7(4), 803–16.

Richardson, A. & Ream, E. (1996) The experience of fatigue and other symptoms in patients receiving chemotherapy. *European Journal of Cancer Care*, 5 (Suppl. 2), 24–30.

Rinck, G.C., van den Bos, G.A.M., Kleijnen, J., de Haes, H., Schade, E. & Veenhof, C.H. (1997) Methodologic issues in effectiveness research on palliative cancer care: a systematic review. *Journal of Clinical Oncology*, 15, 1697–1707.

Ripamonti, C.B. & Bruera, E. (1997) Dyspnea: pathophysiology and assessment (review). *Journal of Pain and Symptom Management*, 13, 220–32.

Robbins, M., Jackson, P. & Prentice, A. (1994). *Palliative Care Provision in the South West*. Health Care Evaluation Unit, University of Bristol.

Robbins, M. (1998) *Evaluating Palliative Care; Establishing the Evidence Base*. Oxford University Press, Oxford.

Roberts, D.K., Thorne, S.E. & Pearson, C. (1993) The experience of dyspnea in late-stage cancer. *Cancer Nursing*, 16(4), 310–20.

Roth, A.J. & Breitbart, W. (1996) Psychiatric emergencies in terminally ill cancer patients, *Hematology/Oncology Clinics of North America*, 10(1), 235–9.

Rousseau, P. (1995) Hospice and palliative care. *Mosby Year Book; Disease a Month*, 41(12), 771–844. Mosby, St. Louis.

Rowland, K.M., Loprinzi, C.L., Shaw, E.G. *et al.* (1996) Randomised double blind placebo-controlled trial of cisplatin and etoposide plus megastrol/placebo in extensive stage small cell lung cancer. *Journal of Clinical Oncology*, 14, 135–41.

Sadovska, O. (1997) Department of palliative care in Bratislava and the development of the palliative care movement in Slovakia. *Support Care Cancer*, 5(6), 430–4.

Sales, E. (1991) Psychosocial impact of the phase of cancer on the family: an updated review. *Journal Psychosocial Oncology*, 9, 1–9.

Saunders, M. (1983) Careers: Macmillan nursing. *Nursing Mirror*, 157(7), 56.

Schneider, D., Adler, D. L. & Gotsch, A. (1996) Hospice in New Jersey: 20 years of progress. *New Jersey Medicine*, 93(11), 41–6.

Schonwetter, R.S. (1996) Care of the dying geriatric patient. *Clinical Geriatric Medicine*, 12(2), 253–65.

Seale, C. & Kelly, M. (1997) A comparison of hospice and hospital care for people who die: views of the surviving spouse. *Palliative Medicine*, 11, 93–100.

Simons, J.P., Aaronson, N. Vansteenkiste, J.F., te Velde G. *et al.* (1996) The effects of medroxyprogesterone acetate on appetite, weight and quality of life in advanced-stage non-hormone-sensitive cancer. *Journal of Clinical Oncology*, 14, 1077–84.

Simons, J.P. (1997) *Cancer Cachexia*. Dissertation, University of Maastricht, the Netherlands.

Sirkia, K., Hovi, L., Pouttu, J. & Saarinen-Pihkala, U.M. (1998). Pain medication during terminal care of children with cancer. *Journal of Pain and Symptom Management*, 15(4), 220–26.

Slevin, M.L., Plant, H, Drinkwater, J. & Gregory, W.M. (1988) Who should measure quality of life, the doctor or the patient? *British Journal of Cancer*, 57(1), 109–12.

Smets, E.M., Garssen, B., Schuster-Uiterhoeve, A.L. & de Haes, J.C. (1993) Fatigue in cancer patients. *British Journal of Cancer*, 68(2), 220–24.

Smets, E.M., Garssen, B., Bonke, B. & de Haes, J.C. (1995) The Multidimensional Fatigue

Inventory (MFI); psychometric qualities of an instrument to assess fatigue. *Journal of Psychosomatic Research*, **39**(3), 315–25.

Smets, E.M.A. (1997) *Fatigue in cancer patients undergoing radiotherapy.* Dissertation, University of Amsterdam.

Spencer, D.J. & Daniels, L.E. (1998) Day hospice care – a review of the literature. *Palliative Medicine*, 12, 219–29.

Spiegel, D., Bloom, J.R. & Yalom, I.D. (1981) Group support for patients with metastatic cancer. A randomised prospective outcome study. *Archives of General Psychiatry*, 38, 527–33.

Spiegel, D. & Bloom, J.R. (1983) Group therapy and hypnosis reduce metastic breast carcinoma pain. *Psychosomatic Medicine*, 4, 333–9.

Spiegel, D., Sands, S. & Koopman, C. (1994) Pain and depression in patients with cancer. *Cancer*, 74, 2570–8.

Spiller, J.A. & Alexander, D.A. (1993) Domiciliary care: a comparison of the views of terminally ill patients and their family care givers, *Palliative Medicine*, 7, 109–15.

Sprangers, M.A. & Aaronson, N.K. (1992) The role of health care providers and significant others in evaluating the quality of life of patients with chronic disease: a review. *Journal of Clinical Epidemiology*, **45**(7), 743–60.

Sprangers, M.A. & Aaronson, N.K. (1996) Kwaliteit van leven bij evaluatie van kankertherapie. *Ned Tijdschrift Geneeskunde*, **140**(12), 646–9.

Spreeuwenberg, C. (1997) Palliatieve zorg (Palliative care). *Medisch Contact*, 52, 149.

Steen van der, L.E.H.M. (1997) Is de zorg naar wens, meneer? Een onderzoek naar de bruikbaarheid van een meetinstrument binnen de Nederlandse palliatieve zorg (*Is care acceptable? Study of the validity and reliability of an instrument in the Dutch palliative care*). Doctoraalscriptie (Masters thesis), Faculty of Health Sciences, Maastricht University, Maastricht.

Steiner, N. (1997) Symptom control and palliative care. *Revue Medical Suisse Romande*, **117**(3), 165–73.

Stephens, R.J., Hopwood, P., Girling, D.J. & Machin, D. (1997) Randomised trials with quality of life endpoints: are doctors' ratings of patients' physical symptoms interchangeable with patients' self-ratings? *Quality of Life Research*, **6**(3), 225–36.

Sterkenburg, C., King, B. & Woodward, C. (1996) A reliability and validity study of the McMaster Quality of Life Scale (MQLS) for a palliative population. *Journal of Palliative Care*, **12**(1), 18–25.

Stetz, K.M. & Hanson, W.K. (1992) Alterations in perceptions of care giving demands in advanced cancer during and after the experience. *Hospice Journal*, 8, 21–34.

Stiefel, F., Kornblith A. & Holland, J. (1990) Changes in the prescription patterns of psychotropic drugs for cancer patients during a 10 year-period. *Cancer*, 65, 1048–53.

Stone, P., Hardy, J., Broadley, K., Tookman, A., Kurowska, A. & Hern, R.A. (1999) Fatigue in advanced cancer: a prospective controlled cross-sectional study. *British Journal of Cancer*, **79**(9/10), 1479–86.

Strang, P. (1992) Emotional and social aspects of cancer pain. *Acta Oncologica*, **31**(3), 323-6.

Sykes, N.P. (1991) A clinical comparison of laxatives in a hospice. *Palliative Medicine*, 5, 307–14.

Sykes, N.P. (1996) An investigation of the ability of oral naloxone to correct opoid-related constipation in patients with advanced cancer. *Palliative Medicine*, 10, 135–44.

Tamarin, A., Milocchi, F., Tolley, K., Vaglia, A., Marcolini, F., Manfrin, V. de Lalla, F. (1992) An economic evaluation of home-care assistance for AIDS patients: A pilot study in a town in northern Italy. *AIDS*, **6**(11), 1377–83.

Tchekmedyian, N.S., Hariri L., Siau J. & Tait, N. (1990) Megastrol acetate in cancer anorexia and weight loss. *Proceedings of the American Society of Clinical Oncology*, 9, 336.

Teunissen, S. & Blink van den, J. (1997) Centrum voor ontwikkeling van palliatieve zorg; vernieuwen is de moeite waard. *Medisch Contact*, 52(31), 159–60.

Tierney, A. J., Anderson, J., King, M., Lapsley, I. & Llewellyn, S. (1994) Measuring the cost and quality of palliative care: a discussion paper. *Palliative Medicine*, 8, 273–81.

Toverud Severson, K. (1997) Dying cancer patients: the choices at the end of life. *Journal of Pain and Symptom Management*, 14, 94–9.

Trotter, J.M., Scott, R., Macbeth, F.R., McVie, J.G. & Calman, K.C. (1981) Problems of the oncology outpatient: role of the liaison health visitor. *British Medical Journal*, 282, 122–4.

Trzepacz, P.T, Baker, R.W. & Greenhouse, J. (1988) A symptom rating scale for delirium. *Psychological Research*, 23, 89–97.

Tsamandouraki, K., Tountas, Y. & Trichopoulos, D. (1992) Relative survival of terminal patients in home versus hospital care. *Scandinavian Journal of Social Medicine*, 20(1), 52–4.

Twycross, R.G. (1991) Why palliative medicine? *Henry Ford Hospital Medical Journal*, 39(2), 77–80.

Twycross, R.G. (1993) Symptom control: the problem areas. *Palliative Medicine*, 7 (Suppl. 1) 1–8.

Twycross, R. (1997) *Introducing Palliative Care*, 2nd edn. Radcliffe Medical Press, Oxford/New York.

Vachon, M.L.S., Kristjanson, L. & Higginson, I. (1995) Psychosocial issues in palliative care: the patient, the family, and the process, and outcome of care. *Journal of Pain and Symptom Management*, 10, 142–50.

Vainio, A. & Auvinen, A. (1996) Prevalence of symptoms among patients with advanced cancer: an international collaborative study. Symptom Prevalence Group. *Journal of Pain and Symptom Management*, 12, 3–10.

Varni, J.W., Thomson, K.L. & Hanson, V. (1987) The Varni/Thompson Pediatric Pain Questionnaire: 1. chronic musculo-skeletal pain in juvenile rheumatoid arthritis. *Pain*, 28, 27–38.

Ventafridda, V., De Conno, F., Vigano, A., Ripamonti, C., Gallucci, M. & Gamba, A. (1989) A comparison of home and hospital care of advanced cancer patients. *Tumori*, 75, 619–25.

Ventafridda, V., Ripamonti, C., de Conno F. & Tarburini, M. (1990) Symptom prevalence and control during cancer patients' last days of life. *Journal of Palliative Care*, 6(3), 7–11.

Ventafridda, V., de Conno, F. & Blumhuber, H. (1993) Palliative care in Europe. *Journal of Pain and Symptom Management*, 8(6), 369.

Vinciguerra, V., Degman, T.J. & Sciortino, A. (1986) A comparative assessment of home versus hospital comprehensive treatment for advanced cancer patients. *Journal of Clinical Oncology*, 4, 1521–8.

Viney, L.L., Walker, B.M., Robertson, T., Lilley, B. & Ewan, C. (1994) Dying in palliative care units and in hospital: a comparison of the quality of life of terminal cancer patients. *Journal of Consulting Clinical Psychology*, 62, 157–64.

Voltz, R., Akabayashi, A., Reese, C., Ohi, G. & Sass, H. (1997) Organization and patients' perception of palliative care: a cross-cultural comparison. *Palliative Medicine*, 11, 351–7.

Von Gunten, C.F., Neely, K.J. & Martinez, J. (1996) Hospice and palliative care: program needs and academic issues. *Oncology Huntington*, **10**(7), 1070–4.

Von Roenn, J.H., Cleeland, C.S., Gonin, R., Hartfeld, A.K. & Pandaya. K.J. (1993) Physicians' attitudes and practice in cancer pain management: a survey from the eastern oncology cooperative group. *Annals of Internal Medicine*, 119, 121–6.

Wakefield, M. & Ashby, M. (1993) Attitudes of surviving relatives to terminal care in South Australia. *Journal of Pain and Symptom Management*, 8, 529–38.

Waller, A.C. (1996). *Handbook of Palliative Care in Cancer*. Butterworth-Heinemann, Boston.

Walsh, R. (1987) *Death: always a threat … sometimes a reality*. Jones and Bartlett, Boston.

Ward, S.E., Goldberg, N., Miller-McCauley, V., Mueller, C., Nolan, A., Pawlik-Plank, D. *et al.* (1993) Patient-related barriers to management of cancer pain. *Pain*, 52, 319–24.

Webber, J. (1994) Palliative care. A model response. *Nursing Times*, 90(25), 66–8.

Weitzner, M.A., McMillan, S.C. & Jacobsen, P.B. (1999) Family caregiver quality of life: differences between curative and palliative cancer treatment settings. *Journal of Pain and Symptom Management*, **17**(6), 418–28.

Weitzner, M.A. & McMillan, S. (1999) The caregiver quality of life index – cancer (CQOLC) scale: revalidation in a home hospice setting. *Journal of Palliative Care*, **15**(2), 13–20.

Wenk, R. (1993) Argentina: status of cancer pain and palliative care. *Journal of Pain and Symptom Management*, 8(6), 385–7.

WHO (1990) Cancer pain relief and palliative care. *Report of a WHO Expert Committee*. WHO, Geneva.

WHO (1998) *Cancer Pain Relief and Palliative Care in Children*. WHO, Geneva.

Wilkie, D.J. & Keefe, F.J. (1991) Coping strategies of patients with lung-cancer related pain. *Clinical Journal of Pain*, 7, 292–9.

Winningham, M.L., Nail, L.M., Burke, M.B., Broody, L., Cimprich, B., Jones, L.S., Pickard-Holley, S. & Rhodes, V. (1994) Fatigue and the cancer experience; the state of the knowledge. *Oncology Nursing Forum*, 21(1), 23–6.

Wit de, R. & van Dam, F.S. (1997) Verbetering kwaliteit pijnbestrijding met pijn instructie programma (Improvement in pain management quality with pain instruction program). *Kanker (Cancer)*, 21, 12–14.

Wit de, R., van Dam, F., Hanneman, M., Zandbelt, L., van Buuren, A., van der Heijden, K., Leenhouts, S., Loonstra, S. & Abu-Saad, H.H. (1999a) Evaluation of the use of a pain diary in chronic cancer pain patients at home. *Pain*, 79, 89–99.

Wit de, R., van Dam, F., Abu-Saad, H.H., Loonstra, S., Zandbelt, L., van Buuren, A., van der Heijden, K. & Leenhouts, G. (1999b) Empirical comparisons of commonly used measures to evaluate pain treatment in cancer patients with chronic pain. *Journal of Clinical Oncology*, 17, 1280–87.

Wit de, R., van Dam, F., Loonstra, S., Zandbelt, L., van Buuren, A., van der Heijden, K., Leenhouts, G. & Abu-Saad, H.H. (2000a) The Amsterdam pain management index compared to eight frequently used outcome measures to evaluate the adequacy of pain treatment in cancer patients with chronic pain. *Pain* (in press).

Wit de, R., van Dam, F., Loonstra, S., Zandbelt, L., van Buuren, A., van de Heijden, K., Leenhouts, G., Duivenvoorden, H. & Abu-Saad, H.H. (2000b) *European Journal of Pain*, (in press).

Wolfe, J., Grier, H.E., Klar, N., Levin, S.B., Ellenbogen, J.M., Salem-Schatz, S., Emanuel, E.J., & Weeks, J.C. (2000) Symptoms and suffering at the end of life in children with cancer. *The New England Journal of Medicine*, 3(20), 326–33.

Working Party on Clinical Guidelines in Palliative Care (1997) *Changing Gears –
Guidelines for managing the last days of life*. National Council for Hospice and
Specialist Palliative Care Services, London.

Working Party on Clinical Guidelines in Palliative care (1998) *Guidelines for Managing
Cancer Pain in Adults*. National Council for Hospice and Specialist Palliative Care
Services, London.

Yang C. & Kirscling, J.M. (1992) Exploration of factors related to direct care and outcomes of care giving: caregivers of terminally ill older persons. *Cancer Nursing*, 15,
173–81.

Zigmond, A.S. & Snaith, R.P. (1983) The hospital anxiety and depression scale. *Acta
Psychiatrica Scandinavia*, 76, 361–70.

Zimmer, J.G., Groth-Juncker, A. & McCusker, J. (1984) Effects of a physician-led home
care team on terminal care. *Journal of the American Geriatrics Society*, 32(4), 288–92.

Zimmer, J.G., Groth-Juncker, A. & McCusker, J. (1985) A randomised controlled study of
a home health care team. *American Journal of Public Health*, 75(2), 134–41.

Further Reading

Anderson, J., George, R.J., Weller, I.V., Lucas, S.B. & Miller, R.F. (1991) Complications of treatment for cryptosporidial diarrhoea (clinical conference) *Genitourinary-Medicine*, **67**(2), 156–61.

Blesch, K., Paice, J., Wickham, R., Harte, N., Schnoor, D., Purl, S., Rehwalt, M. & Koop, P. (1991) Correlates of fatigue in people with breast or lung cancer. *Oncology Nursing Forum*, 18, 81–7.

Carter, J. (1996) Can hospice care be provided to people who live alone? *Home Health Nurse*, **14**(9), 710–6.

Ford, G. (1993) A palliative care system: the Marie Curie model. *American Journal of Hospital Palliative Care*, **10**(4), 27–9.

Ford, G. (1996) Marie Curie Cancer Care and palliative care research – a personal view (editorial). *Palliative Medicine*, **10**(3), 181–4.

Glaus, A. (1994) Fatigue and Cancer; indivisible twins? A comparison between cancer patients, patients with diseases other than cancer, and healthy people. *Pflege*, **7**(3), 183–97.

Grey, D., MacAdam, D. & Boldy, D. (1987) A comparative cost-analysis of terminal cancer care in home hospice patients and controls. *Journal of Chronic Diseases*, **40**(8), 801–10.

Gurfolino, V. & Dumas, L. (1994) Hospice nursing. The concept of palliative care. *Nursing Clinics of North America*, **29**(3), 533–46.

Hughes, S.L., Ulasevich, A., Weaver, F.M., Henderson, W., Manheim, L., Kubal, J.D. & Bonarigo, F. (1997) Impact of home care on hospital days: a meta analysis. *Health Services Research*, **32**(4), 415–32.

Kearsley, J.H. (1986) Cytotoxic chemotherapy for common adult malignancies: 'the emperor's new clothes' revisited? *British Medical Journal of Clinical Research and Education*, **293**(6551), 871–6.

Kellar, N., Martinez, J., Finis, N., Bolger, A. & von Gunten, C.F. (1996) Characterization of an acute inpatient hospice palliative care unit in a US teaching hospital. *Journal of Nursing Administration*, **26**(3), 16–20.

Kristjanson, L.J. (1989) Quality of terminal care: salient indicators identified by families. *Journal of Palliative Care*, 5, 21–8.

McGrath, P.A. (1990) *Pain in Children: nature, assessment, and treatment*. Guilford Press, New York.

Mercadante, S. & Trizzino, G. (1997) The SAMOT supportive care programme in southern Italy. *Support Care Cancer*, **5**(1), 5–8.

NCHSPCS (1996) *Palliative Care in the Hospital Setting*. National Council for Hospice and Specialist Palliative Care Services, London.

Rousseau, P. (1994) Hospice care (letter; comment). *Journal of American Medical Association*, **272**(10), 767.

RCPCH (1997) A guide to the development of children's palliative care services. *Report of the joint working party of the RCPCH and Association for Children with Life-Threatening Conditions and their Families.* Royal College of Pediatrics and Child Health, London.

Seale, C. (1991) A comparison of hospice and conventional care. *Social Science and Medicine*, 32, 147–52.

Seale, C.A.-H. & Addington-Hall, J. (1994) Euthanasia: why people want to die earlier? *Social Science and Medicine*, 39, 647–54.

Sontag, M.A. (1996) A comparison of hospice programs based on Medicare certification status. *American Journal of Hospital Palliative Care*, 13(2), 32–41.

Steiner, N. & Luchsinger, V. (1997) Mobile team for palliative care in Geneva. *Revue Medical Suisse Romande*, 117(3), 249–53.

Tamburini, M. & Rosso, S. (1992) A therapy impact questionnaire for quality of life assessment in advanced cancer research. *Annals of Oncology*, 3, 565–70.

Thompson, I. (1984) Ethical issues in palliative care. *Palliative Management of Far Advanced Disease.* Oxford University Press, London.

Tol-Verhagen van, C., Zuurmond, W.W.A. & Steijns, O. (1997) Kuria: vier jaar palliatieve zorg in Amsterdam; een complementaire zorgverlening (Kuria, four years palliative care in Amsterdam, supportive care). *Medisch Contact*, 52(31), 157–8.

Verwey, K.H. (1997) Profits through principles: Netwerk voor palliatieve zorg voor terminale patienten Nederland (Network for palliative care for terminal patients in the Netherlands). Network, Utrecht.

Wenk, R., Alegre, C. & Diaz, C. (1993) Palliative care hotline in Argentina (letter). *Journal of Pain-Symptom Management*, 8(3), 123–4.

Willems, D. (1997) Wie doet wat in de palliatieve zorg thuis; verslag van een conferentie (Who does what in home palliative care; conference report). *Medisch Contact*, 52, 31 Jan., 167–8.

Zylicz, Z., Borne van den, H.W. & Bolenius, J.F.G.A. (1997) Intramurale zorg voor terminale patiënten in hospice Rozenheuvel; evaluatie door nabestaanden en huisartsen, (Intramural care for terminal patients in Hospice Rozenheuvel; evaluation by family survivors and family physicians). *Medisch Contact*, 52(5), 154–6.

Index

Evidence-Based Palliative Care
Across The Life Span